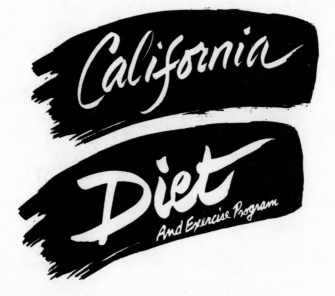

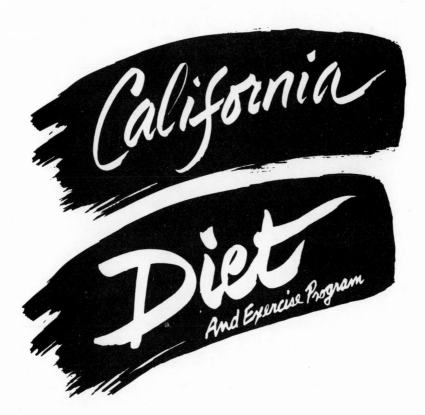

California Diet

And Exercise Program

DR. PETER WOOD

Anderson World Books, Inc.
1400 Stierlin Road
Mountain View, CA

For Christine, Loretta
and Montmorency

CONTENTS

ACKNOWLEDGMENTS _____ 9

INTRODUCTION _____ 11

PART ONE:

PLAY MORE, EAT MORE, WEIGH LESS

   1. What Makes a Good Weight-Loss Plan?_____ 17

   2. Getting Out of the Diet Rut_____ 33

   3. The California Diet and Exercise Program _____ 51

   4. Is There Life After Weight Loss? _____ 69

PART TWO:

LEARNING TO PLAY AGAIN

   5. Exercise as Play, Not Work _____ 81

   6. How To Become a Playful Person _____ 89

   7. Link Your Eating to Your Play_____ 115

   8. The Health Benefits of Play _____ 119

PART THREE:

INGREDIENTS FOR A HEALTHY DIET

   9. Carbohydrates, Fat, Protein _____ 145

  10. Vitamins, Minerals, Fiber_____ 159

  11. Dietary Villains? _____ 167

  12. The California Foods_____ 175

PART FOUR:

THE CALIFORNIA DIET EAT AND PLAY PLANS

Introduction _____ 194

Eat and Play Plans _____ 195

Calorie Plans _____ 203

Exchange Lists _____ 231

Recipes _____ 251

Play Plans _____ 272

References _____ 279

About the Author_____ 288

CONTENTS

ACKNOWLEDGMENTS _____ 9

INTRODUCTION _____ 11

PART ONE:

PLAY MORE, EAT MORE, WEIGH LESS

  1. What Makes a Good Weight-Loss Plan?_____ 17

  2. Getting Out of the Diet Rut_____ 33

  3. The California Diet and Exercise Program _____ 51

  4. Is There Life After Weight Loss? _____ 69

PART TWO:

LEARNING TO PLAY AGAIN

  5. Exercise as Play, Not Work _____ 81

  6. How To Become a Playful Person _____ 89

  7. Link Your Eating to Your Play_____ 115

  8. The Health Benefits of Play _____ 119

PART THREE:

INGREDIENTS FOR A HEALTHY DIET

  9. Carbohydrates, Fat, Protein _____ 145

  10. Vitamins, Minerals, Fiber_____ 159

  11. Dietary Villains? _____ 167

  12. The California Foods_____ 175

PART FOUR:

THE CALIFORNIA DIET EAT AND PLAY PLANS

Introduction _____ 194

Eat and Play Plans _____ 195

Calorie Plans _____ 203

Exchange Lists _____ 231

Recipes _____ 251

Play Plans _____ 272

References _____ 279

About the Author_____ 288

ACKNOWLEDGMENTS

I am very much indebted to Darlene Dreon, M.S., M.P.H., R.D., who devised the calorie plans and recipes in this book, and also contributed a great deal to the nutritional philosophy presented here. Her assistance in preparation of the manuscript was invaluable.

Ms Patti Mathis and my wife, Christine, provided excellent stenographic support for this project.

It has been a pleasure working with Richard Benyo and Ray Hosler during the preparation of *The California Diet and Exercise Program*.

Finally, my thanks to many colleagues at the Stanford Heart Disease Prevention Program for countless discussions over the years of the principles put forth in this book.

INTRODUCTION

"The solution to our national overweight problem is to encourage people to eat more."

Of course, this is a provocative statement. But consider the following observations:

• How much you eat has little relationship to how much you weigh.

• Americans seem to be eating less nowadays, but are not losing weight.

• The most active people in our society are not only slim — they eat more than the overweight.

For years we have been giving overwhelming attention to the left-hand side of the weight control equation:

$$Energy\ in = Energy\ out$$

Now we need to give equal attention to the energy-expenditure-side of the equation; and in the process you may well "eat more but weigh less." *The California Diet* is intended for the moderately overweight adult. I have recruited the best available scientific information to win the weight control battle. Many respected scientists and medical authorities have devoted their careers to the subject of weight control, and they have much to say; yet many people seeking to lose weight are misled into taking advice from . . . almost anyone else! We must give up limitless faith in witless weight-loss schemes and devices; cease being the "blind and deaf tenants of our bodies;" reject the "Speed of Light Diet" as the old, hopeless "get rich quick" scheme.

The need for increased playfulness among our overweight population is the central, overriding theme of this book. Why say "play" rather than exercise? Because I define "play" as the sort of exercise that is enjoyable, and that is the type of exercise we should promote; we are more likely to do it, and to adopt it as part of our lives. Don't think of your personal energy as electrical energy, or energy from oil or gas, to be conserved. North Americans are great hoarders of personal energy, and many have waistlines to prove it. Be wasteful! Stand, don't sit; walk, don't stand; run, don't walk! Don't save steps, spend them. Be energetic! Why? Because that's what slim people do — and it's fun.

Besides being the key to easy weight loss and permanent weight control, regular play also brings with it a host of health benefits, from improved heart performance to decreased inclination to smoke. Play tones the muscles, and as you lose weight you need good muscles to maintain your new, lighter body. Adequate time for play should be sacred to everyone — built into union contracts, fought for like liberty.

But what of "dieting," counting calories? This book will present calorie restriction as a temporary measure for losing accumulated fat, to be done only in conjunction with increased play; it is *not* to become a desirable way of life, in which "taking small bites," "hiding food" and the like are permanent features.

There are many disadvantages and some dangers in the permanent low-calorie approach to weight control, whereas there are many advantages associated with the hearty eating approach. Don't let the diet books con you into the confining, low-calorie lifestyle. Out with the old "sit still, watch the screen and eat your celery" life for the overweight. In with the "dance and play, build bridges and eat hearty" life that nature intended.

You will find in *The California Diet* a concern for the *quality* of the food we eat, during weight loss, and forever. Recent research indicates that many natural foods are beneficial to health, and may help to ward off the major chronic diseases of the day — heart disease and cancer. There is much more to learn, and as the German monk and scholar St. Thomas à Kempis said:

"All perfection in this life hath some imperfection mixed
with it: and no knowledge of ours is without darkness."

But at this time it is certainly prudent to eat heartily of fresh fruits and vegetables, for many of which California is the major supplier.

This is an era of "downsizing" — small cars, smaller houses, less steel, less oil, less rubber. It sounds like bad news for the industries concerned, but wait; there is good news for many industries. In the future we will need more healthy food, more facilities for play.

In *The California Diet and Exercise Program* you will notice a particular concern for the older person. Medical science has given us more years of life, added to our fifties, sixties and seventies. Why? Well, not to spend it in the doctor's waiting room, I hope.

Many older people are inactive, overweight and poorly nourished. We need to work on this rapidly increasing problem with a sense of urgency. The magnificent machine of medical science, so spectacularly successful in prolonging life, needs to be wound up again and set to improving quality of life. But we already know many of the answers, and they do not involve drugs or surgery: They are simple things we must do for ourselves. According to Joseph Califano, formerly Secretary of Health, Education and Welfare, "We [Americans] must replace our prevailing ethic of expensive self-indulgence with an ethic of rigorous personal responsibility. Government cannot enforce it. Doctors cannot administer it like a drug. We face a choice between taking increased responsibility for our own health and continuing the present wasteful sick-care system, with its staggering toll in dollars, wasted lives and grief."

And as Richard S. Schweiker, formerly Secretary of Health and Human Services, said, "By taking five simple steps, by not smoking, by using alcohol in moderation, by eating a proper diet and getting the proper amount of exercise and sleep, a 45-year-old man can expect to live 10 or 11 years longer than a person who does not make these choices.

"We must convince people how to take control of their own health, how to adopt habits that can make trips to the doctor less frequent. Prevention should be in the minds of every American, and at the heart of every health care institution."

If *The California Diet* helps us to move in the direction of a slimmer, healthier and happier life, it will have achieved its purpose.

PART ONE: PLAY MORE, EAT MORE, WEIGH LESS

PART ONE: PLAY MORE, EAT MORE, WEIGH LESS

1. What Makes a Good Weight-Loss Plan?

The man or woman today who is overweight, and wishes to do something about it, has a problem. Later I shall try to define "overweight," which is not as simple as you might think; "overfat" is a more accurate, if less familiar word. And there are many reasons why a certain human body is considered to be "overfat." The medical view of "fatness" is not fixed; it evolves in the light of new medical evidence; it depends to some extent on your sex and your age; and society's views on what constitutes an appropriate, aesthetically pleasing, or sexy body vary with the society and with the decade.

The Problem

But large numbers of people — certainly many tens of millions in the United States alone — are clearly overweight by almost any contemporary standard and, more importantly, they want to do something about it. I'll rephrase that more realistically: They are itching to do something about it, and downright frustrated that their efforts to date have not been successful. This is the problem: frustration. Now, there is another, smaller group of frustrated people: those professionals — physicians and scientists — who work in the area of weight control and nutrition. They look on in dismay at an American population that is heavier than ever, and given to many deplorable dietary habits. The problem has arisen, and persists, largely because of an avalanche of misinformation. Myriads of erroneous words are printed on miles of misleading paper with gallons of garrulous ink, all masquerading under exotic titles, from the Chinese Gooseberry Weight-Loss Program to the Timbuktu Diet. At the same time, megabucks travel through the mails to purchase miraculous elixirs and incredible devices that will melt fat magically or take off pounds in microseconds. Unfortunately, as almost everyone really knows, this vast, circuitous exercise usually brings the overweight person back one year later close to where he started: a few pounds heavier, a few more dollars out of pocket and . . . a little more frustrated.

Taking Care of Yourself

The late John Knowles said:

"The next medical breakthrough is the patient taking responsibility for his own health."

There is a tremendous, overdue need for the overweight public to take a critical look at programs offered — usually sold — to them. We need to evaluate, to spurn transparent nonsense. "Let the buyer beware" is never more true than when the customer is purchasing "weight control." What Knowles was saying is that people need to use their own sense and judgment, carefully nurtured at vast expense by our public education system, to improve their own health and quality of life. In many areas we cannot rely on "society" to do this for us: The billboard encourages us to smoke; we have some 470,000 physicians in the United States — but concomitantly a large, frustrated overweight population. Each of us must develop a critical approach to proposals and advice that affect the most important aspect of our lives — the health of ourselves, our families and our friends.

If we plan to buy a car, we all ask simple questions before we plunge in: number of cylinders? automatic transmission? miles per gallon? This evaluation process may take days or weeks, and the enquiry may get quite complex. It is unfortunately true that many people will plunge into a weight-loss program with virtually no enquiry; it's as if the car buyer didn't notice that the vehicle has no wheels, the engine is missing, or the brakes don't work. Not surprisingly, when the buyer gets in to take a trip the weight-loss car doesn't go anywhere. Or if it does move, it may be downright dangerous. Of course, we wouldn't tolerate this situation with new cars, but we seem quite tolerant of ineffective, sometimes hazardous, new weight-loss programs. You see what Knowles was getting at. Since our society is rightly reluctant to "ban" books and ideas, we need to be particularly critical and on guard.

What Makes a Good Weight-Loss Plan?

I have worked in the health promotion field for many years. In the past 10 years I have seen many people — millions across the United States — successfully lose weight and maintain weight loss in spite of the barrage of misleading diet information to which they have been exposed. They achieved this result by ignoring all this information. It was the very fact that they *didn't* read the diet books that enabled them to lose weight! There is an important lesson to be learned from this group of men and women who successfully bucked the trend and lost weight while the average American continued to put it on, engrossed in his diet book. The plan presented here, which you are about to read, incorporates much of what we have learned by scientific methods in recent years about weight loss and nutrition. Of course, the plan "tells you what to do." But to be true to Knowles I want to explain the plan, invite your comments and answer questions as we go along. You should know why this plan is likely to work for you. You should be a partner in the weight-loss program, not simply an overweight person following instructions. You should automatically ask a series of questions every time you encounter a new weight-loss program, challenge it for scientific worth, search it for logic.

Don't you need profound scientific insight and years of training to do this? Many of the points are simply common sense, and others require some knowledge of modern findings in weight control. Let's look together at 10 characteristics of a good plan to lose weight and keep it off. If a proposed plan is lacking in any one feature, it will be worthless, or at least have serious drawbacks. I do not propose to make a detailed critique of the many diets, familiar and obscure, that have come and gone — or of the ones that are still very much with us. But I think you will find that most of these diets clearly fail on several of the following points, and you will be "uncertain" about several others. Almost every popular plan fails in at least one important respect. In proceeding in this way we can examine what we'd like to see in a weight-loss plan, what really matters to us; and in the process we can work toward an ideal solution — *The California Diet and Exercise Program.*

Safe. This is the paramount feature, surely, of any acceptable diet or weight-loss plan. And yet many approaches turn out to be unsafe. A number of diets provide calories almost entirely in the form of protein, with very little of the main energy sources — carbohydrate and fat. Subsistence on such "liquid protein" diets and other high-protein diets frequently leads to feelings of malaise and weakness, as the body notices the complete absence of its usual fuel supply and is forced to metabolize the protein, producing waste products that lead to uncomfortable feelings. But things can get worse than this for the few unfortunate dieters who suffer electrolyte imbalance and, occasionally, disturbances of the heart rhythm — even death. And there are several other unfortunate consequences. For this reason, diets that provide large amounts of protein but are very low in carbohydrate are frowned upon by medical authorities, and some have been banned. A diet that allows "all the lean meat you can eat," but very little else, may sound attractive, and will probably result in considerable weight loss — until you feel so sick you have to give up, or worse. Really, this is *not* a fun way to lose weight!

Many other diet plans are simply very low in total calories. At levels below about 1000 calories per day, it is very difficult to obtain sufficient nutrients to meet the body's needs. Multiple vitamin and mineral capsules can replace some of the missing nutrients, but probably not all. Long periods spent on very low-calorie diets, without proper replacement of essential nutrients, can be dangerous. Remember that people who have gone on fasts — oftentimes for political reasons — drinking only water, typically suffer permanent eye damage from vitamin deficiency, and die within 50 to 70 days. Be on the safe side and avoid *very* low-calorie diets.

Quite a variety of weight-reduction "aids," taken by mouth, enjoy popularity yet are not safe. Amphetamines, stimulatory drugs that effectively decrease appetite, have been decried by medical authorities for many years. They have several undesirable effects (dry mouth, irritability, insomnia) and are addictive. It's not worth losing weight and acquiring a "habit."

There seems to be no end to the ingenuity of purveyors of diet aids, who will produce almost anything salable that can be used to circumvent the reasonable, natural, inexpensive road to a good body weight. A recent arrival is the "starch blocker." These tablets contain the protein phaseolamin, extracted from kidney beans, which interferes with the normal enzymic digestion of starches in the small intestine. The starch, only partly digested, continues on to the colon where it is set upon by bacteria, producing gas that can cause a number of problems — cramps, nausea, diarrhea. There must be a better way to lose weight, short of prejudicing your social life with abdominal cramps and flatulence!

Another approach involves deceiving your body into believing it has been fed when no calories are entering the system. Capsules of glucomannan, a Japanese root extract, swell from water absorption to form a gel that fills the stomach, creating the sensation of fullness and thereby reducing appetite. Sucrose polyester (SPE) resembles fat and can be incorporated into the diet. But it is not absorbed, and so gives the sensation of eating fat, without providing calories. In certain circumstances these preparations may be useful in promoting initial weight loss, for instance in extremely obese people. But they have not yet been extensively tested. I suspect that in the end it will prove unwise, if not impossible, to fool Mother Nature in this way.

Other treacherous or futile routes to your desired weight range from jaw wiring to exercising in rubber suits. You name it, they sell it! So, if your jaws are wired closed, you can only drink through a straw: great for the weak-willed but what happens if you have to throw up one day? You may choke! And the rubber running suit routine will give a spectacular demonstration of how much sweat you *should* be evaporating as you run. But it all collects inside your suit! You may overheat and collapse!

Well, this is probably enough to make my point. Whatever else we do, let's be sure the plan we adopt is safe.

Effective. The sheer number of weight-loss plans in existence testifies to the inadequacy of most of them. True, some overweight people have persevered and have undergone significant weight loss, are happy about this and never look back. We shall study some of these "winners" later in the book to learn what they did right. But millions of other people embark on weight-loss programs with high hopes, only to find, once again, that they don't work. So, look out for indications that the program "won't work."

Look for unreasonable claims. "Lose 10 pounds in five days" is ridiculous. You cannot lose fat (which is what you want to lose) that fast. You are unlikely to lose 10 pounds of *anything* in five days; but if you do, most of it will be water. You can't go on losing water at that rate, so your weight loss will rapidly slow down, which will be discouraging. Soon your weight loss slows to a crawl, even though you are still on the diet. Your body is adapting to less food! Many weight-loss plans result in considerable loss of body water in the first week, so do not be deceived; you don't want to lose body water, just fat. And a *fat* loss of three to four pounds per week is just about the most you can *possibly* lose (short of surgical removal!); and even that is a much faster rate than is advisable, as we shall see later.

Programs that "melt fat away while you sleep," or "speed up metabolism many times" are immediately suspect, and fail the "effectiveness" test.

There is another major reason why many weight-loss programs are ineffective. Perhaps, if adhered to for a long time, they would work. But they are too demanding, too restrictive, too unpleasant, so the dieter quits and, again, the diet doesn't work. Watch for diets that emphasize one or two foods: the raisin diet or the asparagus diet. Does it sound likely that you would live happily predominantly on one or two foods, rejecting all others, for any length of time? For most people the answer is "no," and the diet fails. Any diet plan that is going to put you on fewer than 1000 calories for more than a few weeks is likely to fail. You simply get too hungry because you are trying to lose weight too fast. So you eventually give up.

Plans that are too fast, too ambitious or make ridiculous claims will usually fail. Like plans to double your money in a month, they are too good to be true. You can see them a mile off.

Permanent. Most people who bother with a weight-loss plan at all have in mind a new body form for themselves, not for a week or a month, but as a permanent feature of their lives. And yet, for those plans that are initially effective, the dieter approaches — may even reach — the promised land, but then relapses and drifts back to being overweight. Because the brief period of looking-good-in-a-swimsuit was enjoyable, and clearly the diet did work, let's try again. And again, and again. In fact the diet *didn't* work, not by my definition anyway, because it lacked any real permanence. This repeated battle to get down to some desired weight, won for a week but then lost again, is familiar to millions. It has been called "the rhythm method of girth control."

How do we detect a plan that will probably fail because it lacks permanence? After all, the books don't come stamped "Lacks Permanence" on the front cover. Look for a diet plan that puts you on a calorie-restricted diet *temporarily* — not permanently. People don't like permanent diets, so they quit. Look for a plan, later in the book, that tells you what to do when you've lost weight. So many diet books leave you dangling, several sizes smaller but unsure of what to do next. You get the impression that you either go on dieting forever, until you fade away to nothing and can use yourself as a bookmark, or you quit, gain it all back (because your life hasn't really been changed by the literary experience) and then start all over again at Chapter 1.

Treating yourself like a metabolic yo-yo is not a good idea. There is a strong feeling among weight-loss experts that people who have gained, lost, gained, lost, through many cycles become particularly resistant to permanent weight loss, so it's better not to put yourself through this depressing experience. There is also reason to believe that some of the physiologically harmful effects of overweight operate particularly when weight is being actively gained, rather than when weight is steady. The process of weight gain may adversely affect your blood cholesterol, for instance, and so indirectly worsen the risk of atherosclerosis (hardening of the arteries) and heart attack.

A good diet plan should lead the dieter gently to a new, permanent healthy way of life when the weight-loss phase is over. A plan that heads you into the sunset on a permanent "low-calorie" diet, counting calories forever, is not a good solution. In my view, low-calorie diets (i.e., diets that contain fewer calories each day than you need for an active life) should be used sparingly and therapeutically to achieve loss of accumulated fat; they should *not* be prescribed as a permanent, desirable, modern, with-it, and thoroughly admirable way of life. Life — especially California life — requires food! More about this vital subject later.

Scientific. There is a romance about witchcraft and mysticism that appeals to us all. And it is nice to dream of success without struggle, and weight loss without effort. But let's face it, our best hope of success in a rather difficult task like permanent weight reduction is likely to be based on good science. Some weight-loss plans are based on poor science or no science, and many on witchcraft. Another way to look at the question is this. All of us have spent some of our hard-earned dollars on medical research, sponsored by the federal government. And it produces results, at first buried in the scientific literature, then gradually applied for the public good. Some very good minds have grappled with the problem of weight loss. Now, I am not pretending that we know all about weight control: It is a complex, difficult subject. But there are many guiding principles that really do contribute to solving the problem — your problem.

As a taxpayer you should say "I've spent good money on this work. I want to know what you experts have to tell me about safe, effective, permanent weight loss." Doesn't this make more sense than embracing witchcraft and taking the word of the latest "witch" who has persuaded a publisher to push her diet book with its sexy title? (I apologize for this sexist remark, and gladly include all diet wizards in this indictment.) So, look for reason in your diet plan, and beware of exotic fruits masquerading as science.

Wards Off Chronic Diseases. Since 1900, a profound and astonishing change in America's health has taken place. Life expectancy has increased greatly, although the *oldest* people in the population today are probably no older than were the oldest people in 1900. Investment in public health and medical research has paid off handsomely, in this way: deaths in infancy (diphtheria, measles, whooping cough) and in early adulthood (tuberculosis, pneumonia), removed huge numbers of young individuals from the population in those days, before they had really gone very far in life. Today, a death before the age of 50 is relatively unusual, and is often the consequence of accident, homicide or suicide — not disease. Disease prevention — remarkable in its degree and rapidity — has given life in huge packages of years to relatively young people, and has enabled them to live to be middle-aged, or old. A visit to one section of a churchyard (1870-1940) reminds us of the frequency and acute sadness of young people "taken before their time" by infectious disease.

But we are still mortal, and we still get sick. In fact "health care costs" continue to escalate at an alarming rate. Probably those benefactors, with names increasingly unfamiliar to their countless beneficiaries, who virtually eliminated diphtheria and typhoid, believed at the time that sadness, infirmity and medical expense would be greatly reduced in America by their noble efforts. Well, not altogether so; because chronic diseases such as heart disease, cancers, lung diseases and arthritis have afflicted those children and young adults who had been "saved" from the ferocious infectious diseases of the past. So now we have a generally more mature population, becoming progressively older year by year, and causing great concern to those responsible for Social Security retirement benefits. Many men will now live into their late seventies, and many women well into the eighties; but frequently they will be disabled earlier on by chronic disease, removed from the work force but unable to enjoy retirement. And so it becomes of great concern and interest to us all to avoid or minimize or at least postpone the ravages of the chronic diseases of older age. It is not so much a question any more of avoiding premature death (these are predominantly diseases of middle and old age); but it is a question of preserving health, vitality and happiness into the fifties, sixties and seventies, the years that many of us would not have seen at all 80 years ago. This subject has been eloquently discussed by Fries and Crapo in *Vitality and Aging.*

Now what has all this to do with weight control? Well, first, today's overweight people are part of the population with many more years of life expectancy, the same as everyone else. A successful, permanent weight-loss plan is for them an important part of the campaign to reduce risk of chronic disease, and to improve quality of life in the older years. High blood pressure and diabetic tendencies, with their sad consequences, are worsened in millions of people simply because they remain overweight. But my main point here is to ensure that in the process of losing weight by your weight-loss plan, you don't inadvertently increase your risk of chronic disease later.

There are two important parts of a weight-loss plan to examine: the nutritional composition of the diet you will eat, and the type and amount of exercise you will get on your plan. Both of these areas will be looked at in detail later in this book, but for the purposes of this review of desirable characteristics of a weight-loss plan, look for these features, with the diseases they may help to avoid or alleviate, in parentheses.

Diet

- Relatively low in total fat (some cancers, atherosclerosis)
- Relatively low in refined sugar (dental caries)
- Moderate alcohol (cirrhosis, some cancers)
- Low in saturated fat (atherosclerosis)

- Low in cholesterol (atherosclerosis)
- Low in salt (high blood pressure)
- Relatively high in carotene (some cancers)
- Relatively high in fiber (atherosclerosis, diverticulosis, some cancers)

Activity

- Promotes regular exercise (atherosclerosis, osteoporosis)
- Promotes aerobic exercise (atherosclerosis)
- Promotes flexibility (arthritis)
- Promotes not smoking (several cancers, emphysema, bronchitis)

A weight-loss plan would fail this test if it disregarded these vital dietary and activity areas. The longer the plan keeps you on a program where the diet is promoting chronic diseases, and exercise is ignored or given lip service only, the more deficient the plan is. It is as if the proponents of some weight-loss plans were concerned only with the removal of body fat, and were oblivious to the increased risk of heart attack, for instance, that accompanies long-term use of the plan. Of course, everybody, fat or thin, should pay attention to his food intake, exercise habits and smoking behavior. By no means do we know everything about the association of these factors with chronic diseases; but there is overwhelming evidence that a prudent diet, regular exercise and not smoking are as important to our health today as improved sanitation and diphtheria immunization were for our parents and grandparents.

So, look too for features of a weight-loss plan that will ward off — not promote — chronic diseases. How many weight-loss plans do you know that pay no attention to your future health? As George Herbert said: "The buyer needs a hundred eyes, the seller not one." **Promotes Fitness.** We have touched on fitness, but it deserves further discussion. Some weight-loss plans manage to fill 300 pages with no mention of physical activity. More typically, a page or two among hundreds of pages on diet points out that the weight loss, and later weight maintenance process, will probably go better if the dieter also takes some exercise. In fact, calorie intake — as food — and calorie expenditure — as metabolic and muscular activity — are the two equally important, balanced poles of the process that is life.

It is curious that one of the two poles has been absurdly overemphasized relative to the other in the area of weight control. It is as if we were trying to control the amount of gas in the gas tank of a vehicle by devoting all our efforts to changing the amount, frequency and type of fuel added, but were totally oblivious to whether we are adding gas to the tank of a motor bike or a large truck, and to how far and how fast the vehicle travels. The rate at which fuel is used — our physical activity level — clearly has to be as important a factor in weight control as the rate at which fuel is added — our dietary intake. Perhaps it is a feeling that the overweight will be discouraged by the prospect of exercising more that has led to this lopsided treatment of weight control. But it has also been well demonstrated that the overweight are discouraged by the prospect of eating less over long periods of time. I believe a modern, balanced picture should be presented, and the person wishing to lose weight should participate in the plan decided upon.

There are two major reasons why you should look for an exercise component in your weight-loss plan. The first is that the plan is much more likely to work that way; here we get back to the "effectiveness" test. As we shall see in later chapters, there is much modern scientific evidence to show that weight *maintenance* (the key to lifelong desirable weight) is much easier for active people than for sedentary people. So you look for an exercise component in any proposed plan simply because the plan is much more likely to be effective.

The second point is that regular exercise promotes physical fitness and physical fitness frequently brings with it a host of benefits that you may not get from weight loss alone:

• Improved performance (from climbing stairs to sex)
• Improved heart function and respiratory function
• Lower resting pulse rate
• Improved blood cholesterol picture
• Denser bones
• Lessened need to smoke
• Regularity
• Improved sleep
• Improved mental outlook

These are some of the most important factors that add up to an improved quality of life — especially during those extra years in the fifties and beyond that so many people will now live through. So why settle for weight loss alone, when you can have physical fitness too? And remember, physical fitness does not mean becoming an Olympic athlete. You don't even have to become a jogger (although you probably could, with benefit). All sedentary people can obtain benefits from small but regular amounts of exercise that should be fun. In fact, I'm going to refer to our sort of exercise as play, which is what it should be. We're going to get into this enthusiastically later in the book. Meanwhile, when looking over a weight-loss plan, check it out for fitness promotion — and insist on a play plan.

Leads to Eating More — Not Less! That sounds pretty preposterous, doesn't it, a weight-loss plan that encourages you to eat more than you are eating now even though you're overweight? But when we study the issue carefully, we'll see that this should be a goal of a successful, long-term plan. We just learned that very active people have a much easier time maintaining their weight than sedentary people. In order to remain active, you need more fuel — more food calories. So, logically, the best-placed people to maintain their desirable weight are people who have to eat a lot to remain very active. We can see this relationship in operation in the real world. Groups of people who have desirable body weights and good-looking figures, especially after 30, include: tennis players, cyclists, runners, people who walk a lot, people always on the go. How much do they eat? Active, lean people typically eat rather large amounts of food, and often *much* more than sedentary but overweight people. So "eating a lot" doesn't necessarily have any relation to being overweight; in fact, generally the reverse is true: The overweight usually don't eat much! They do, of course, eat too much relative to their low activity level. But how much is "too much?"

The typical overweight American at age 50 has put on one to two pounds of fat each year since he was 20 years old. So at 50 he is 30 to 60 pounds overweight — and it shows. But a gain of one to two pounds of fat each year means eating only 10 to 20 calories too much each day on average, or no more than a quarter of a small banana! In other words, the calorie imbalance that is making the overweight person steadily, inexorably fatter (with occasional unsuccessful attempts at dieting thrown in) is actually exceedingly small. But the lean, active person is successfully processing much larger amounts of food; and remaining slim effortlessly. "It's their metabolism," you say, and you're right. But why not learn from this how to change your metabolism: Become active and eat more! If we don't recognize that overweight people, in successfully becoming slim, will be eating the same as when they were fat, or often more, then we have a problem, because this will inevitably happen. We should anticipate it.

There is one other interesting point about eating more. Several long-term scientific studies now agree in indicating that individuals who go on to suffer heart attacks are more likely to have been eating *less,* years earlier, than similar people who remained well. putting it it another way, eating more seems to predict *fewer* heart attacks, in the same way that low blood cholesterol levels predict less heart attacks. We don't know precisely why this is. Perhaps it is the stepped-up activity level that often accompanies increased food intake that is actually protective. And if we have to choose, I think we should opt for a higher calorie intake, in the same way that we should choose to have a lower cholesterol level.

We are beginning to fashion our ideal weight-loss plan along these lines: effective but safe loss of body fat initially, successfully maintained over the long haul in a program that keeps us slim, active, and eating more.

Gradual. We live in a time-urgent world, a world of instant puddings and precipitous weight loss. I admit that claims for producing very large weight losses in a very short time have proved quite attractive to the overweight. There is a constant contest: lose up to six pounds in 10 days; five pounds in one week; 14 pounds in two weeks. As we have learned, most of this loss, if it occurs at all, is loss of water. Inevitably, a spectacular weight loss in the first two weeks of the plan rapidly slows and may stop altogether. Most experts agree that a true loss of body fat of one to two pounds of fat per week is the fastest you should go. But when this loss is slow but sure, you soon overtake the spectacular losses of the water-loss diets:

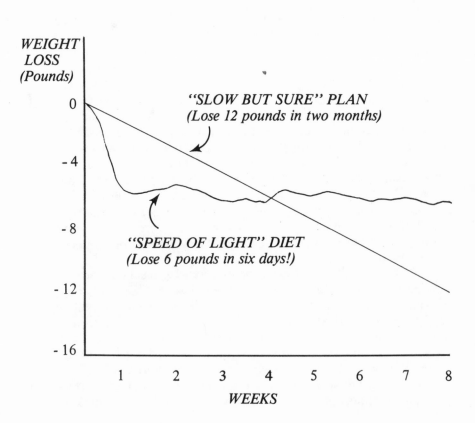

If you are 30 pounds heavier than you'd like to be, at 45 years of age, remember that it probably took 20 years for the extra fat to accumulate. So it's only reasonable to allow some months, perhaps a year, to return to where you were. And since at the same time we want to return your active play level back to where it used to be when you were younger — and beyond — it will also take time for your muscles to gradually accustom themselves to a more active life. Proceeding too fast will lead to aching muscles and the false conclusion that you're past playing anymore! But when you proceed gradually, you will be astonished how far you can go with weight loss and with play.

So don't be deceived by impossible claims of very rapid weight loss. Look for gradualness in a weight-loss plan, one of the hallmarks of success.

Inexpensive. I wonder if there is any relation between the money spent on a weight-loss plan and the weight actually lost? We really don't know, but I doubt it. Perhaps money will buy success for people who are very much overweight, and need to lose 80 pounds or more. Professional assistance is indicated for extreme obesity, and can often be effective, but it will cost money. For those of you with a goal of moderate to minor weight loss, let's look at the balance sheet.

A successful weight-loss diet will not call for low-calorie intake, and it won't be exotic either. Generally, healthy but available foods are recommended. An emphasis on fresh fruits may increase food costs a little, but this will be more than offset by savings on reduced intake of red meat, eggs and some dairy products. A healthy weight-loss diet is not an expensive diet. Later, when you are leaner but eating more, your grocery bill may rise somewhat. But remember that those extra calories are best provided largely by carbohydrate, which generally means grains, vegetables and fruits — foods less expensive than meats and dairy products.

Isn't all this extra play going to be expensive? It needn't be. The type of play that will help your diet plan the most involves inexpensive activities: walking, cycling, swimming, jogging and the like. Of course, you can spend money on expensive clothes and memberships in clubs and spas, but this will only help if your plan is basically sound, and generally it is unnecessary. Most expensive weight-reduction equipment is promoting the wrong sort of play. Machines that pound or massage will do very little to help you lose weight. A bicycle is an excellent investment, and although a stationary bicycle is okay, it's less fun (stationary bicycles are not gregarious, and thus not very useful for meeting other people and having fun). More about equipment later; meanwhile, the purchase of good-fitting running shoes (to walk or jog in) and a good warm-up suit is probably worth all the other equipment put together, and can be yours for less than $150.

Live-in programs or fat farms for weight loss? They're invariably expensive, and probably only useful for people who just won't do anything about their weight unless led by the hand. Whether the dollars invested are converted to pounds permanently lost depends on the weight-loss plan presented. If it is basically unsound, by the criteria we have developed, then it won't help in the long run. If the program is sound during the live-in period, but cannot be "exported" to the home situation and practiced there permanently, then weight lost will be regained rapidly.

The spectacular examples of satisfactory and lasting weight loss in the last 10 years are characteristically groups of people who changed their lifestyles of their own accord, who reasoned it out for themselves. They may have joined cycling clubs or running clubs, and they usually own a bicycle or a tennis racket, and they quite often buy new running shoes. But if you ask them, they won't associate their new figures with the expenditure of large amounts of money. So, the cost of a weight-loss program is no guide to its effectiveness.

Enjoyable. Now we have come full circle from safety to enjoyment. And both are crucial. "Being on a diet" is one of the least enjoyable activities, as anybody who has tried it will tell you, so perhaps you think it's asking a lot to enjoy it. But obviously if you *do* enjoy the plan, or at least parts of it, you are more likely to stick with it, right? And if the plan is gradual, that makes it more likely to be enjoyable than if it is abrupt and painful. And a calorie-reduced diet done in moderation is less painful than a very low-calorie diet, which makes you feel bad, and lethargic. Additionally, isn't a plan that allows you gradually to eat more, until you may be eating more than you did in the past, more enjoyable and encouraging than a permanent "low-calorie" approach? Don't people basically enjoy eating? And don't people who play and exercise regularly all agree on one thing: they feel better! And isn't one cardinal rule of enjoyment, the first step, to "feel better?" And isn't progressively losing weight, getting out to play with other people, feeling fitter and younger, isn't that enjoyment?

So what's all this about weight-loss programs being purgatory? Some no doubt are, but they don't have to be. Look for a program that gives you something to look forward to: a fit body and good meals, not a lifetime on and off diets. The successful weight losers I keep referring to found the whole process enjoyable and, of course, that's why they were successful. After all, if it's not enjoyable, it probably won't work.

Synthesis

The critical features of a good weight-loss plan are listed below:

• Safe
• Effective
• Permanent
• Scientific
• Wards off chronic diseases
• Promotes fitness
• Leads to eating more — not less
• Gradual
• Inexpensive
• Enjoyable

The overweight participant should emerge from a weight-loss program healthy, happy, lighter and, most importantly, confident of what to do next — and forever — to stay that way.

The plan you will find in Chapter 3, *The California Diet and Exercise Program*, is based on all of these principles. It is designed for men and women who are mildly to moderately overweight. People who are very much overweight (80 pounds or more above their ideal weight, as calculated on pp. 54, 55) will obtain some helpful guidelines from this plan, but they will benefit more fully from professional advice.

2. Getting Out of the Diet Rut

WHY THE CALIFORNIA DIET AND EXERCISE PROGRAM?

The title of my diet plan suggests a program conceived and practiced in California.

Why "California"? Well, the program originated in California and it has been unconsciously practiced by millions of active Californians as they have played and eaten their way to health and slimness in the last 10 years. The idea of "Eating More But Weighing Less" seems crazy enough for California — a state that specializes in crazy ideas that everybody eventually adopts. And the healthy foods frequently come from the fertile valleys of California.

Why "Diet"? To most of us, diet means a program to lose weight. But, of course, the word "diet" is much more general than that. A Random House dictionary definition says: "A particular selection of foods, especially as prescribed to improve physical condition or to cure or prevent disease." And that is precisely the sense in which we use it in *The California Diet*. This definition says nothing about "fewer calories" or restricting anything. *The California Diet* is a weight-loss plan, but just as important it is a lifestyle, designed to improve physical condition, and to cure or prevent disease. Conscientiously followed, it will do just that. As you embark upon *The California Diet*, you are overweight, out of shape and not very playful. When you leave it, one year later, you will be slimmer, fit, playful and free to enjoy California's foods.

The breakthrough here concerns our perceptions of why people become fat and stay fat, and what they should do about it. The idea that being overweight is caused and sustained by eating inordinately large amounts of food has been with us for many centuries, and dies hard. We picture Shakespeare's corpulent character, Falstaff, hanging out at the Boar's Head tavern, eating heartily. Shakespeare knew that being grossly overweight was not good for the health, but

33

he blamed the condition on overeating, as Prince Hal says to Falstaff:

"Leave gormandizing; know the grave doth gape
For thee thrice wider than for other men."

Falstaff's exercise habits are never mentioned, although he did seem to do a lot of sitting — and sleeping — in the Boar's Head. And when given a "charge of foot" to take to the wars, Falstaff protests "I would it had been of horse (whores)." He has a predilection for strumpets, but also prefers to ride a horse, rather than walk. Our preoccupation with the calorie input side of the diet equation even shows itself in the word "obesity," from the Latin "Ob," (over) and edere (to eat).

Our ideas are changing, and none too soon! We now know that we cannot consider diet without exercise, or exercise without diet, if we are to make any sense of either. They go together like income and expense, profit and loss, ham and eggs. They are two ends of the spectrum — energy in, energy out. A studied neglect of the expenditure side of the ledger along with inspecting the income side in minute detail from all angles, has led to our curious beliefs about the cause and cure of overweight.

Perhaps the half-truth, that "you have to do an enormous amount of exercise to burn off one meal" has been most responsible for the neglect of exercise — of play — as a powerful factor in weight control. It *is* true that the human body is magnificently efficient, and can travel on foot almost 50 miles on one pound of fat. But we can do a lot of playing in one year! I prefer to look at it this way: Most overweight people are putting on only a few pounds a year — say five pounds. This is enough to make them extremely overweight by middle age. Now *The California Diet* has a set of Play Plans to make your exercise easy and fun. They are very gradual and, in fact, the first month is so easy it's absurd. But if we add up all the extra calories you will use on this easy plan, we get a total for the year of 61,500 calories, or 17½ pounds of fat. So our overweight person can stop the five-pound weight gain and lose 12½ pounds of fat by becoming more playful — and we haven't even talked about dieting yet! So I'd rephrase the pessimist's view to read: "You can get a large amount of weight loss by adopting an easy, enjoyable play program."

Let's look at some of these questions in more detail to understand what a modern "diet" should look like.

Eating Little, Resting Often and Growing Fat in America

The proportion of American adults who are "overfat" has been put at anywhere from 30 percent to 90 percent, depending on the author and criteria used. Even if we are quite conservative in our estimate, one of every four adult Americans can afford to lose fat, for health and cosmetic reasons, to be able to play more easily, to have more fun. There are subgroups of overweight people who fall into three categories:

- Under age 18
- Clearly overweight as children
- Extremely overweight — 80 pounds or more over "ideal" weight.

I will not include these groups in our discussion. I believe that they can benefit from the ideas and the plans presented in *The California Diet*; but these are special cases, and I recommend that people in these categories work with a physician or weight-control specialist to achieve permanent weight loss. But I still have an audience of 30 million to 50 million adults who are now moderately overweight, but were not always that way. My discussion is with them.

If a scientist wants to understand a problem, he often uses one or both of two methods:

- The comparison method
- The time course method.

For instance, if he wants to know what to do about pollution in a large city, he might compare a small, unpolluted town with that large city. How do they differ? What pollutants does each have, and how much? What sort of factories and industries does each have, what sort of residents? This is the comparison method, and it gives a lot of information. But, if he had the time and resources, our scientist might try to trace the evolution of a small, unpolluted town into a large, polluted city. He could do this by looking at historical records of a large city from its start as a small town. How did it change? What was the sequence of events? Which factories arrived first? Which pollutants appeared and in what order? He might even do a prospective study, in which he looks closely at one particular small town and follows it as it grows over the years, and becomes polluted: He studies the history of a large city. This time course method gives much more information about how the small town and the large city came to be different.

If a scientist wishes to look at 50 million overweight Americans, he has these two methods available. He can study overweight people and see how they differ from slim people living in the same population, of the same sex and age (the comparison method). He can also look back 10, 20, 30 years and observe the way today's overweight people used to be, and what happened to them (the time course method). He might even follow individual slim young people until they become overweight, middle-aged adults; he would learn a lot, but then he would have to be very patient, and quite long-lived.

Now, it turns out that we do have a lot of information about the overweight, gained scientifically at considerable expense — your expense and my expense, because the majority of such work is done with federal funding. Do people who devise weight-control plans make use of this information? Are they even aware of it? In many past instances, and for many of the best known, most devoutly followed, hallowed diets, the answer to both questions is "no." Too much of the author's time was spent in the food section of supermarkets, or in the test kitchen; too little time was spent in the medical library! In recent years some of the scientific facts have been published in a few good, popular books (see Reference section under Chapter 2 heading). Let's look at some of the major facts and use them to tailor a weight-loss plan that can work.

Comparison Studies. A number of studies have indicated that overweight people tend to be less active than normal-weight people. In some instances this is visually obvious: We less often see overweight people engaging in the more vigorous sports such as running, cycling or racquetball. Of course, there are exceptions: Some overweight people run, but they are rapidly becoming slim; and some slim people take little exercise, but some of them are becoming overweight. If we study groups of people practicing various sports in a dedicated way (soccer, swimming, running, tennis), as has been done on numerous occasions, we almost always find the active group to be slimmer, to have a lower percentage of body fat and to be closer to "ideal" weight than is the average, rather sedentary U.S. population of the same age and sex. So, it is clear that slimness and exercise go together, and that fatness and the sedentary life go together.

That isn't surprising. You can "run off fat." Notice how your dog slims down when he goes on a week-long hiking trip with you, because he's dashing around all the time? But what does the comparison method tell us about the food intake of fat people compared to thin people? Fat people eat more than slim people, you might say. Everyone thinks that; look at Falstaff. But the evidence doesn't show that to be true. Measuring precisely what people eat is difficult because of the expense, time and inconvenience involved. And people who are overweight may be a little reticent about their eating habits while being studied. In spite of these research problems, it is quite clear that overweight people do not eat considerably more than comparable slim people, except in a few unusual groups. On the whole, the reverse is true. For example, in a study of large numbers of London male civil servants it was found that the fatter men generally ate rather *less* than the slimmer men. The classic studies of Jean Mayer have indicated that except in the case of the extremely overweight, the slim tend to eat *more* than the fat. Another interesting comparison study involved many pairs of Irish brothers. One of the pair, who lived in Ireland, was found on average to weigh less but to eat *more* than his brother, who was now a resident of Boston.

Our group at the Stanford Heart Disease Prevention Program has compared middle-aged runners (jogging 40 miles per week) and tennis players (10 hours singles play per week), of both sexes, with average, randomly selected men and women. Steve Blair and coworkers showed that the runners were not only leaner than the sedentary groups, but also ate considerably more. The same was true for the tennis players in a study by Paul Vodak and coworkers.

Calories Consumed per day

Runners	
Men (34)	2959
Women (27)	2386
Tennis Players	
Men (25)	2726
Women (25)	2417
Sedentary Controls	
Men (73)	2450
Women (49)	1490

Of course, the comparison here is quite extreme, between "average" people and very active athletes (male and female) in middle age. But both groups are going about their business, earning their living; the exercisers are not a race apart, they simply spend 3 to 10 percent of their time in a favorite vigorous activity. At the same time they are much slimmer, but eat considerably more. The case of the tennis playing women is particularly striking: They are reporting eating about 62 percent more than their more sedentary, heavier "average" counterparts.

Time Course Studies. In the past 80 years Americans, on average, have been getting fatter — they have drifted farther away from their "ideal" weights, and their bodies now contain relatively larger proportions of fat. The prevalence of "obesity" in the population is generally agreed to have almost doubled since 1900. Again, we might expect that the consumption of energy in food (calories eaten) would have increased since 1900, accounting for the increased amount of obesity. But records indicate that average intake of calories per day has actually *declined* considerably since the early 1900s. The decrease in calorie consumption appears to have been continuing during the last decade, as shown by national food consumption surveys conducted in the United States in 1965 and again in 1977 and 1978. During this 12-year period, measured calorie consumption dropped for all age groups and both sexes. Okay, so we had a big, successful dieting campaign on a national scale? People really ate less and lost weight, right? Well, that's not altogether true. No doubt people ate less, but national surveys of weight and height conducted during this "dieting" period give no indication that the American public lost weight overall. Dr. Mark Hegsted, administrator of the Human Nutrition Center of the United States Department of Agriculture (USDA) at the time the findings were released, said: "We are as big and fat as we ever were, and obesity may be gaining on us. About the only interpretation possible at this time would be that Americans are becoming increasingly sedentary."

Another fascinating finding of these surveys relates to the fate of food produced. It is estimated that the United States produces a food supply of about 3500 calories per person per day. About 2900 of these food calories enter the home each day in the grocery bag. However, only 1800 to 1900 calories per day are actually eaten. There are two points of interest. First, where does the enormous amount of uneaten food go? Its cost and volume is vast. Presumably some of it feeds our non-human domestic friends; some is destroyed in cooking; but most of that 1000 missing calories per capita per day goes to waste. It amounts to vast acreages of corn, enormous herds of cattle, gargantuan flocks of turkeys, gigantic orchards, all in the garbage. Seems a shame, really, doesn't it — all that work and money down the drain? *The California Diet* will show you how to resolve the problem, help the farmer, lose weight, eat more, feel better and play!

For a final example of the time course approach to understanding what has been happening in America, I will tell you the result of a one-year study done by my colleagues and me at Stanford University, which looked at changes in exercising individuals over time (see Reference section). Eighty-one middle-aged but quite sedentary male faculty and staff took part. Forty-eight were assigned at random to start an exercise program in which jogging regularly was encouraged over the next year. Neither group was deliberately encouraged to diet, lose weight or change diet; they were merely monitored in these respects. The remaining 33 were assigned to remain as sedentary controls. We made careful measurements of miles logged by the exercisers during the year (of course, they didn't all manage exactly the same amount of jogging), of their body fat loss or gain during the year, and of the amount of food they typically consumed. When the study was over, we found that the men who had done the most jogging had lost the most body fat — hardly surprising. The men who did the most jogging showed the biggest increase in food calories — not really surprising, except to those who believe that exercise suppresses appetite. The controls changed very little. But another finding was that the jogging men who lost the most fat also increased their food intake the most. They were indeed eating more but weighing less within one year. Of course, they were also playing more! It is unreasonable to conclude from this study that the solution to America's creeping overweight problem is to eat less, when the most successful weight losers were those who *increased* their food intake, and the least successful were those who didn't! Remember, none of these men were asked to lose weight; they were simply asked to adhere to a jogging program.

Let's look at what happens quite often to young people, of good body weights, as they set sail on the ocean of American life. A lot changes between age 20 and age 50. Typically, many of the more energy-consuming activities — dancing, tennis, staying up late — are set adrift. There just doesn't seem time for them anymore, what with the kids and the work piled up at the office: "I mean, honestly, I can't just take off and jog around the block when I am supposed to take a client to lunch, can I?" And so it went, through the unfit 1950s and the sedentary 1960s. For many people, leaving their twenties and entering their thirties and forties meant a lot less fun, a lot less play. Television became a dominant, all-pervading influence. "Watching television," at a cost of two calories per minute, was reportedly America's top leisure time "activity" in 1982, followed by reading a newspaper, which was followed by listening to music at home. "Exercising" was fifth, which, admittedly, is encouraging; and "engaging in sex," which burns more calories than watching television, was way back in 14th position. So, for many people who are middle-aged today, getting older was accompanied by being less active and probably, unless we "do it to television," having less fun and playing less!

During these years our eating habits changed, too. It wasn't that we didn't get dinner invitations, or we couldn't afford to eat; actually, formal meals became more frequent, and we could afford to eat out at restaurants more often as we got older. But frequently we were not so hungry as we used to be. Remember those days when you were 20, and you came home absolutely ravenous! You cooked up two huge cans of spaghetti and then ate three bananas and a glass of milk. When did you last do that? Shame, because satisfying a full-blown appetite is one of life's pleasures. But many people don't feel that hungry very often, and meals are something of a habit. After all, you have to eat. Do you ever feel that restaurants always have the same old stuff? It's just not exciting anymore? But it's your appetite, not the menu, that's at fault. Try hiking for two days without food, and then go to the restaurant. Food will taste much better.

Statistics tell us that the average man and woman in the United States puts on one to two pounds of weight, largely as fat, each year between the ages of 20 and 50, so that is how I calculate my audience of 50 million people who would like to lose 20 to 60 pounds. If we look at the amount of food responsible for weight gain of, say, 1½ pounds of fat per year (or 45 extra pounds by age 50), we go through the following calculation:

$$1½ \text{ pounds of fat} = 1½ \times 3500$$

$$\text{or: } 5250 \text{ calories}$$

$$\text{This is } 5250 \div 365, \text{ or } 14.4 \text{ calories per day}$$

In other words, all it takes is 14.4 calories too much each day for 30 years to store up 45 pounds of fat we don't want at age 50. This amounts to about a fifth of a banana too much each day, for example. So we haven't exactly been gormandizing all these fattening years. The extent of the calorie imbalance is minute, relative to our total daily food intake. In fact, it is so small that it is virtually impossible to describe it, prescribe it, proscribe it or prohibit it.

Returning briefly to the National Dietary Surveys, we find that the average calorie intake of the generally well-padded U.S. population today is not high. It averages about 1900 calories per capita per day, not much different from the food intakes of underdeveloped countries where obesity is rare and malnutrition often a problem.

We Want You to Eat More — and Better!

The scientist, unencumbered by myth and tradition and looking at the evidence, might reasonably conclude that overweight has nothing to do with how much people eat, or he might even interpret the evidence to indicate that those who eat the most are the leanest. As you probably know, high blood cholesterol levels *predict* heart disease and, in the same way, high food intake *predicts* leanness. So moving an individual, or a nation, toward a lower food intake is not likely to be the general cure for our overweight problem, although this may be advisable for some individuals in the short-term.

Let's look at some of the benefits that accompany eating more, rather than following the traditional diet path to perpetually eating less. The catalog is remarkably impressive.

RMR. There is a physiological measurement known as *resting metabolic rate* (RMR). This is the rate at which the body uses energy, measured as calories, when it is essentially at rest, for instance sitting quietly. This resting rate of calorie use ranges from about 1.0 to 1.5 calories per minute. (For comparison, a person running hard may use 20 or more calories per minute). This amount of energy is just keeping the system going, keeping the organs functioning and maintaining body temperature. RMR is rather like a car engine when idling. Although the RMR is a low rate of calorie use, it is very important in relation to whether you are gaining or losing weight, remaining fat or remaining slim. The reason for this is that the RMR operates *all* the time, awake or sleeping. So we can see what effect an *increase* in RMR from 1.0 to 1.2 calories per minute has over a day:

$$0.2 \times 60 \times 24 = 288 \text{ calories}$$

This is the equivalent of walking or running about three miles, but the fat burning is all done at rest. If nothing else changed, a person able to increase his RMR from 1.0 to 1.2 calories per minute would lose 30 pounds of fat in a year!

The reverse is also true. A person who *decreases* his RMR from 1.2 to 1.0 calories per minute would have to walk or run about three miles per day to counteract this fall. Or, if nothing else changed, he would *gain* 30 pounds of fat in a year.

So we can see that the health and welfare of our RMR is a very important matter that is at the heart of weight control. Why has it been absent from countless discussions of diet calories and exercise calories? Probably because the differences in RMR we are talking about — although very important — are small, and so are difficult to measure accurately.

Clearly, this all leads to the question: "What can we do to change our RMR?" Thin people might want to decrease it, fat people to increase it. Many factors influence RMR, including:

• Body size — a large car engine uses more gas even when idling than a small car engine.

• Temperature — it takes more fuel to maintain body temperature when it is cold than when it is not.

- Certain drugs.
- Level of regular exercise — we will come to this later.
- Level of regular food intake.

The level of regular food intake is what we are concerned with now.

The higher your typical food intake, the higher your RMR.
The lower your typical food intake, the lower your RMR.

I hope you begin to see a difficulty emerging for the dieter; it has been referred to as *The Dieter's Dilemma* (see Reference section). As you reduce food intake, your body lowers its fuel use to partially offset the dieting. Here is an extreme hypothetical example:

A fat person reduces calorie intake 288 calories per day by dieting. His body accommodates by lowering RMR from 1.2 to 1.0 calories per minute (although he does not notice this). Nothing else changes. His calorie requirements drop by:

0.2 x 60 x 24 = 288 calories per day

Result: He loses no weight at all!

This sabotaging effect of calorie restriction appears to become more pronounced the greater the degree of calorie reduction (i.e., very low-calorie diets) and the more frequently a person goes on and off diets (the rhythm method of girth control). It is really all very unfair, but that's life. Of course, nature has built in this mechanism for a purpose. People faced with starvation must accommodate in order to survive. Eons ago this was an annual problem for our cave-dwelling ancestors — surviving the winter. More recently, concentration camps and droughts have provided the same desperate conditions. The body is presented with less and less food. It senses that a calamity is approaching. It lowers its RMR accordingly to economize. The population of Leningrad, during the prolonged siege of 1941 to 1944, undoubtedly had very low RMRs, which allowed a proportion to survive. Unfortunately, even if you are quite overweight and can live off your fat for months, your body's reaction to a sudden drop in food is one of alarm: It is going to play it safe and economize by dropping the RMR. The body can't really be expected to know the difference between the first day on the 850-calorie "Arabian Nights Diet" and the first day in Belsen.

I have put this somewhat dramatically to emphasize that an approach to permanent weight control that does not lower the RMR, and preferably increases it, is highly desirable. And that approach is *not* perpetual dieting! So raising your RMR is at the top of the list of reasons that we would like you to eat more!

More Goodies. Provided we eat a sensible diet, it generally follows that "more is better." If we eat more total calories, we eat more food. As we eat more food, we eat more vitamins, more minerals, more carbohydrates, more fiber, more bulk; and there are good reasons (discussed in Part III) to believe that this is good for our health. So again, there are health virtues associated with eating more, not less. An example is nutrient intake in runners. I am often asked by new runners: "Now that I am running a lot, should I eat more vitamins, more minerals, more protein?" Now, as we have seen, runners eat more than sedentary people, so I usually reply: "You already do."

There is another concern of public health here. In spite of the relative prosperity of the United States, there are worries about adequate intake of some nutrients for the country as a whole. There has been concern (at least by some experts) about iron (especially for women), calcium, vitamin C, zinc, selenium, carotene and fiber. The problem is that a substantial number of Americans eat so few calories (e.g., levels of 1400 to 1600 in older women) that deficiencies of some nutrients might easily occur on a poor diet. This again argues against a national policy of encouraging people generally to eat less ("to control weight"), because this can only worsen supposed problems with nutritional adequacy.

Quality of Diet. The watchful reader may comment at this point: "Well, if you say that eating more is good because you will eat more good things in the process, won't you also end up eating more cholesterol, more saturated fat, more salt, and more additives and preservatives, for instance? And aren't these bad for you?" This is a very valid point that must be attended to. There is a hazard that very active people who eat a great deal will select their diet inadvisedly and store trouble for themselves. They may deceive themselves into thinking that diet doesn't matter as long as they are active. The solution: People who are moving toward the benefits of eating more should be assisted in choosing a diet that is deemed nutritious and healthful by nutritionists. *The California Diet* ensures that as you progressively eat more, you eat well — probably much better than you are doing now. This is a public health opportunity we must not miss: As people eat more, we must encourage them to eat better. The public is very receptive to health information at this time — it must be sound. Is your present diet nutritionally sound? If it is a weight-loss diet, does the author know if it's sound?

Constipation. Constipation may sound like a curious subject to bring up now. But the fact is, constipation is an annoying, very common affliction. Some authorities claim that constipation is at the root of other, more serious conditions: hemorrhoids, diverticulosis, even colon cancer. In any event, we are better off without it. What are the causes of constipation? Inadequate exercise is one, to be considered in Part II. Inadequate fiber, inadequate bulk, simply inadequate food is a second, major cause. Why are older, sedentary people plagued by constipation? They tend A) to be inactive and, hence, B) don't eat much, and so C) don't get much bulk. I believe that the human digestive tract was designed to process much more food than the American of the 1980s gives it. We are prisoners of our evolutionary past, and so we have a mechanism to protect us from starvation, which now backfires on the dieter; and also a digestive tract that expects to be fed as if we were running around all day hunting for our food, not sitting all day looking at the computer screen or television. Not only does the system typically get few calories to process, it also gets low-residue food of high caloric density — fat and sugar especially — so that almost everything is absorbed by the time the food gets to the colon, which then has very little to work on. Result: constipation, and infrequent, sad little stools. Moral: Eat more, and eat more fiber! Many people who are overweight say that they "eat like a bird." It's true! But their digestive tract might be heard to complain: "I am the gastrointestinal tract of a full-grown man, not a sparrow. And just 1900 calories a day is, well, ridiculous!"

Calories and Heart Disease. Here is a scientific finding not well known by the public. It turned up in the numerous *prospective population studies* done in the past 30 years. In these, measurements are made of members of a large population, who are then followed for many years to see who develops diseases (such as heart disease) and who dies. The Framingham Study is a famous example in the United States. Such studies have told us that people with high blood pressure or high blood cholesterol levels are more likely to develop heart disease, and to die from it, later in life. So these are "risk factors" for heart disease. What is much less well known is that measurement of food intake has also been done, with the finding in no less than five studies (see Reference section) that people developing heart disease reported eating fewer calories many years earlier than those not developing heart disease. To be consistent, we have to say that regularly eating few calories is a risk factor for heart disease; and we might hypothesize that eating more calories (as with lowering blood pressure or blood cholesterol) will help prevent heart disease. Much remains to be done in this important area of research, but I believe most scientists, in the light of present evidence, would choose to eat more, rather than less, if forced to make a choice. And each day, we are forced to make a choice: We must decide what to eat.

This finding was inevitably regarded as rather paradoxical. After all, eating more suggests gluttony once again, and all that this conjures up (back to Falstaff!). And again, some people were advocating eating less as a national goal "to control weight." What the data are probably telling us is that the people in the studies who were eating more were also *more active,* and *leaner*; and these two attributes accounted for their reduced heart disease rates.

Enjoy! Enjoy! We like to think that behind all our endeavors is the pursuit of happiness. One approach to weight control would be to employ an army of behavioralists to persuade overweight people that they can be perfectly happy eating rather little. They would have a tough job. I would prefer to have the same army turn much of its attention to persuading people to take more exercise, be vital, have more fun. That might be easier. It's really more defensible, at least for most moderately overweight people. If people enjoy eating, are miserable when they can't eat normally, associate so many social and domestic pleasures with eating, why, let 'em eat! To put it more formally, those who would issue the edict 'eat less' will encounter formidable behavioral, psychological and social resistance.

Adherence. Adherence is the technical word for sticking to a weight-loss program. All the evidence is that adherence to most weight-loss programs is dismal. Weight lost with great fortitude and gritting of teeth, by Draconian dieting, is frequently regained in a few months or years. Why? There are two major reasons: (1) As we have seen, dieting tends to be self-defeating, because of its negative influence on the RMR, and so dieters get frustrated; and (2) People like to eat, and don't like to diet, at least not for extended periods, with no hope of return to normal eating.

Farmers and Restaurants. There are some very practical, commercial and industrial implications to *The California Diet.* You will recall that the U.S. agricultural and food production industries can provide about 3500 calories per day per head of the population, but that only about 1900 calories are actually consumed. Perhaps some of my readers are farmers or food-processors or restaurant proprietors. Perhaps you grow the food for *The California Diet* or sell it in a supermarket or serve it in a cafeteria. These are huge industries, they need the business! An interesting consequence of losing weight by *The California Diet* is that you will be helping your neighbor and your fellow worker. Eating less has very negative implications: less fuel, less energy, less action, less vitality, less farming, less business, more empty restaurants. American wheat farmers are having a hard time disposing of their wheat. But wheat, especially whole grain wheat, is a very good food. It's just what you would choose to provide those extra calories in a healthy "eat more" diet. So we could help out the wheat farmers and use the extra energy to move ourselves about, instead of using cars so much, which is certainly what Mother Nature intended us to do with our legs. We would not have to abandon our cars, just use them 10 to 20 percent less, especially for short trips. We would then reduce car accidents, lower gasoline use and improve our balance of payments situation . . .

Conclusion. We got away from physiology at the end of this discussion. But consider this point: Do you think that it is sensible national policy to recommend that Americans eat even less than they are eating now "in order to lose weight?"

EXERCISE: THE "USER-FRIENDLY" WAY TO PERMANENT WEIGHT LOSS

Now that we have examined the numerous advantages of eating more, we know there must be a catch. The catch is that activity level must be increased in those people who should be eating more. As with eating, we are simply talking about moving from an unreasonably, unbiologically low level of activity to a healthy, enjoyable and normal level. As we run down the list of benefits attached to the active, *The California Diet* lifestyle, I think you will agree it is rather a desirable catch.

Use Calories Fast. Any activity, even sleeping, burns fat and uses calories; a kiss uses six to 12. It's all a question of how fast, relative to the rate of replenishing calories via food intake. The Play Plans, in Part IV, tell you what activities use roughly how many calories. But, of course, the more vigorous activities burn fuel faster. Jogging, cycling and swimming are champion fat burners. But remember that if you have the time, a mile walked slowly will use nearly as many calories as a mile run fast — it just takes longer.

Raise Your RMR. Regular exercise leads to an increase in the resting metabolic rate, so that the active person is using calories faster even when not exercising (see Reference section). As we just read, increasing your food intake increases your RMR, too. The two are inevitably intertwined, because increased exercise leads to increased food intake, which leads to increased RMR. But probably there is a relatively acute effect of exercise that operates independently of increased food intake.

There is an hypothesis, known as the "Setpoint Theory," that says an individual tends to hold on to some amount of body fat (the Setpoint) regardless of food intake. With a high setting, the individual is destined to be fat, or at least to have a hard struggle to be slim, and with a low setting the person is destined to be thin. The Setpoint is the amount of fat you tend to store in your body when you have free access to food. The hypothesis also holds that the level of exercise is one of the few ways available to change the Setpoint. In other words, the exercising body likes to be slim, and the sedentary body likes to be fat. Whether or not the Setpoint Theory becomes pollinated into a full-blown theory depends on the amount of effort put into testing it. Another way of looking at the Setpoint is to think of our having a "thermostat" that operates to control our body fat content; it is much more precise and reliable at high rates of calorie flow (high exercise level), but tends to get stuck in the "on" position at low calorie flow (low exercise level), resulting in unbridled accumulation of fat. Very often it seems that the body weight of a very active person is controlled unconsciously, without resort to diets, within very close limits. In my own case, from age 18 to 53 my fully hydrated body weight has never been lower than 119 pounds and never higher than 125.

The Setpoint Theory needs a great deal more research and refinement. Meanwhile, it is clear that everything conspires against the overweight person who remains sedentary.

Lose Heat Faster. As a person increases his exercise level, he tends to lose fat. Fat beneath the skin has a valuable insulating function. This is why successful long-distance swimmers tend to be well padded — they need to keep warm in cold water. Conversely, I am the first to shiver in an unheated swimming pool. The fat person is efficient, conserving; I am wasteful, profligate. But the fat person wishing to lose weight does not want to conserve; he wants to spend, to waste, to burn more fat. The more insulating fat an overweight person loses, the easier it is to keep it off, because he now has to use more fuel to maintain his temperature, and so his RMR rises.

Gain Muscle. Weight loss by dieting without exercise involves loss of muscle as well as fat. This is especially true on very low-calorie diets that are low in protein. In looking for fuel, the body burns part of its muscle as well as its fat reserve. One unfortunate consequence of muscle being burned as fuel is that the amount of muscle left to continue burning fat is decreasing, so that the rate of fat loss slows over time, for this additional reason. But if weight loss is accompanied by increasing exercise level, muscle loss is slowed or stopped. In some cases an exercise program may actually increase muscle mass. This "sparing of lean body mass" during weight loss is very valuable, and is a major advantage of incorporating progressive exercise into a weight-loss program. Of course, it is featured in *The California Diet*.

Move More Mass. The energy cost of walking a mile is usually put at 100 calories. This is an average value for a 155-pound person. If you weighed a lot less, your cost might be only 80 calories. If you weighed a lot more, your cost might be 130 calories. This points out one special advantage of increased exercise for overweight people: The more overweight you are, the more value for money you get from one mile covered. Maybe there is some justice in the overweight world.

Appetite. This is a much argued area in relation to exercise level. "Appetite" is the desire to eat. Some claims say that exercise blunts the appetite, which is probably true immediately after vigorous exercise. Nobody wants to eat a large meal directly after finishing a marathon. But clearly, regular exercise increases the unconscious food intake in the long term, and so presumably *increases* appetite. Newspaper columns that feature doctors who recommend exercise to the overweight because it reduces appetite are well intentioned but usually incorrect: the right advice for the wrong reason. Anyway, who wants to blunt appetites? Satisfying appetites of one sort or another is what life is all about, so why blunt an important appetite if we can lose weight while "eating more?"

Feeling Better About Things. An overweight person probably does not feel all that good about himself. That is why he wants to lose weight. There are feelings of inadequacy, lack of control, loss of a "youthful" figure. Exercise can help enormously here — and has. Mastering an exercise task (swimming 20 laps, or jogging three miles) indicates to the exerciser that he *is* adequate. In the psychological vernacular, his "self-efficacy" is demonstrated. The improved self-esteem, in the physical realm at least, of completing a marathon race has been astonishing in some cases. Many sorts of exercise increase social contacts, and often social support. An overweight woman completing a road race is the recipient of an enormous amount of support from other runners. This is not something that your diet book can do for you. Again, physical activity is still associated with youth, so simply doing it can make your figure *feel* more youthful!

All the Other Benefits. There are a large number of health benefits that accompany physical fitness. These are the subject of Chapter 8, so I won't list them here. But they provide another powerful argument for not short-changing yourself by attempting weight loss without exercise.

Getting Out of the Diet Rut. So, if I were writing a weight-loss program I would put down all these fascinating points in a list and think about them before starting work:

• Slim people often eat more than fat people.
• Conventional dieting leads to reduced resting metabolic rate, frequently sabotaging weight-loss efforts and leading to frustration.
• Conventional dieting reduces muscle mass, which removes energy-burning tissue.
• Low-calorie intakes are associated over the long haul with increased risk of heart disease, poor nutrition and constipation.

- People don't like dieting as a way of life, and tend to resist it.
- Higher levels of food intake are associated with biological, social and economic advantages.
- A long-term food plan should incorporate the best, modern principles of disease prevention.
- Overweight people are often inactive.
- Increased exercise raises resting metabolic rate and often leads to increased food intake.
- Increased exercise tends to increase muscle mass, adding energy-burning tissue, and removing fat.
- Regular exercise provides psychological and social advantages not provided by dieting.
- The active lifestyle brings with it numerous health advantages, independent of weight loss.
- A good weight-loss program should consider the participant's entire future lifestyle, and leave him or her headed resolutely and well informed toward a slim, healthy future.

My consideration of these points led to formulation of an ideal weight-loss plan. The result is Chapter 3. The California Diet and Exercise Program.

3. The California Diet and Exercise Program

At this point we should agree that weight-loss plans can stand rather careful examination, that not all diets are "the same," and that it should be possible to construct a weight-loss plan that emphasizes the good features we have discussed, and discards the bad. The result is not ultra-rapid, flamboyant or exotic: it is scientific, effective and rather unexpected. *The California Diet* is a reasoned appeal for ourselves and our overweight, often frustrated dieting friends to move gradually toward eating more — and playing more.

This chapter gives you the fundamentals of the plan. You will see that the one-year plans presented here incorporate the important features brought together in the first two chapters. The plans cover an entire year because we want to emphasize the gradual approach, to give you time to take off pounds progressively, while you play (*not* "overnight, while you sleep"; this sort of weight loss rapidly returns, "overnight, while you sleep."). A year also allows you time to adopt your new, playful lifestyle gradually, without noticeable strain; and it is your increased play level that is the scientific core of this plan. It is precisely this increased playfulness, combined with a scientific, healthy diet that has accounted for the weight-loss success stories of recent years. The plans package the methods discovered by the active, successful dieters of recent years, and tailor the eating and the play to your own needs.

Here are some general thoughts about these plans.

• They are progressive. You must have faith and see the "big picture." Rewards are built in at planned intervals. As you progress, your eating plans become more liberal; there are new and better foods to eat as the months go by. And the play gets better. We want you to look forward eagerly to the next month when you can graduate to the next play level. Meanwhile, your weight is going in the right direction — down. We'd much rather you lost a few ounces each day, every day, instead of losing six pounds one week and gaining five back the next.

• These plans should be fun! If they are not, concentrate on the play part of the plan. Re-read chapters 5 and 6 on increasing your play activity. Play with other people who want to be more active and lose weight. Playing by yourself is often less fun than playing with a companion. Help each other! We're all in this health game together. We have to take responsibility, as Knowles said. If you can help someone else lose weight, you're almost certain to lose weight yourself. What do you have to do? Be sure you both stay on your play plans!

• Remember that it is impossible to predict *exactly* what weight loss will result from a particular calorie plan and play plan on an individual basis. Unlike most diet books, *The California Diet* presents eight separate plans, to use according to your Maintenance Calorie Intake (that is, the calories we estimate you need to live a rather inactive, unplayful life). But people vary in ways that are impossible to predict. So if your weight loss after you have followed the plan closely for a month or two is considerably *less* than the plan predicts, move to the next *lower* plan (for example, if you are not losing the weight predicted on the 2200 Calorie Plan, move to the 2000 Calorie Plan — your Play Plan won't change). If you are losing weight considerably *faster* than the plan predicts after a month or two, you may be pleased, and can simply stay with the plan. But if you find the plan difficult, not fun, consider going to the next higher plan; for example, if you are losing weight too fast on the 2200 Calorie Plan, move to the 2400 Calorie Plan. If you have read this book, and are impressed with the scientific principles involved in these plans, you will be able to make adjustments yourself — change your eating, change your play, so that your weight is controlled as *you* want it to be. In other words, these plans are guides to get you on the proper metabolic track so that weight control will not be a constant problem. Use them as guides, and modify them with insight.

• Should your physician know about and approve your plan? Physicians have a hard time keeping up with the latest weight-loss diet, and I am sympathetic. The great majority of physicians are likely to be enthusiastic about the underlying principles of *The California Diet*, simply because they incorporate modern, state-of-the-art findings in weight control. If you are not very overweight (not more than 80 pounds above the maximum of your "ideal" weight range) and if you are generally healthy, you are free to proceed with the plan; although it's always a good idea to inform your medical adviser when you plan to change your lifestyle considerably

— and this is what these plans entail. If you are more than 80 pounds above your ideal maximum, or if you have major health problems (heart conditions, lung problems, severe arthritis, diabetes, orthopedic problems, and so on), then you should consult with your medical adviser before beginning these (or any other) weight-loss or exercise plans.

• Should you have minor illnesses (colds, influenza) during your year on the plan, listen to your body and be sensible. A mild cold should mean no interruption. Don't continue with the play plan if you have a fever. Your calorie plan may have to be modified, depending on your physician's instructions, if you are temporarily ill. When you are better, continue from where you left off, or go back a month or two on the plan if you have been completely inactive for more than a week. Don't play harder than feels comfortable!

WHO SHOULD USE THE CALIFORNIA DIET AND EXERCISE PROGRAM?

The California Diet is intended for men and women over the age of 18 who need to lose moderate amounts of weight. To get an approximate estimate of how much weight you can reasonably lose and, indeed, whether you need to lose weight at all, use the following table, which shows the "ideal weights" for men and women of different heights and frame sizes. These are heights in shoes with one-inch heels (for men) and two-inch heels (for women). A range of minimum to maximum ideal weight (in parentheses) is given in each case. So for a man who is 5 feet 8 inches tall in shoes, with a medium frame, the ideal weight is 145 pounds, with a range of 138 to 152 pounds. If in doubt about your type of body frame, use the "medium frame." Find the upper end of the range for you (152 pounds if you are a man 5 feet 8 inches tall) and add 10 pounds. If you weigh more than this amount (162 pounds for our man) you can probably stand to lose some weight. How much weight? You can probably come down to the single ideal weight indicated for you in the table. So our man can lose from his present weight (let's say he now weighs 175 pounds) and achieve 145 pounds, or a weight loss of 30 pounds. Use this table as a guide only. If you are clearly overweight, you will be in little doubt. If you are borderline according to these calculations, you probably need not lose weight for medical purposes, but you may want to reduce weight until you feel happy with the way you look and the way you feel. It is medically important to feel happy about these things anyway!

IDEAL WEIGHT (POUNDS) IN LIGHT CLOTHES* (AND RANGE)

MEN

HEIGHT**	SMALL FRAME	MEDIUM FRAME	LARGE FRAME
4′10″	—	—	—
4′11″	—	—	—
5′0″	—	—	—
5′1″	—	—	—
5′2″	116 (112-120)	124 (118-129)	134 (126-141)
5′3″	119 (115-123)	127 (121-133)	137 (129-144)
5′4″	122 (118-126)	130 (124-136)	140 (132-148)
5′5″	125 (121-129)	133 (127-139)	144 (135-152)
5′6″	129 (124-133)	137 (130-143)	147 (138-156)
5′7″	133 (128-137)	141 (134-147)	152 (142-161)
5′8″	137 (132-141)	145 (138-152)	157 (147-166)
5′9″	141 (136-145)	149 (142-156)	161 (151-170)
5′10″	145 (140-150)	153 (146-160)	165 (155-174)
5′11″	149 (144-154)	158 (150-165)	169 (159-179)
6′0″	153 (148-158)	162 (154-170)	174 (164-184)
6′1″	157 (152-162)	167 (158-175)	179 (168-189)
6′2″	162 (156-167)	171 (162-180)	184 (173-194)
6′3″	166 (160-171)	176 (167-185)	189 (189-199)
6′4″	170 (164-175)	181 (172-190)	193 (182-204)

*For adults aged 18 and above.

**Height in shoes — assume one-inch heel for men and two-inch heel for women.

WOMEN

HEIGHT**	SMALL FRAME	MEDIUM FRAME	LARGE FRAME
4'10"	95 (92-98)	102 (96-107)	112 (104-119)
4'11"	98 (94-101)	104 (98-110)	114 (106-122)
5'0"	101 (96-104)	107 (101-113)	117 (109-125)
5'1"	103 (99-107)	110 (104-116)	120 (12-128)
5'2"	106 (102-110)	113 (107-119)	123 (115-131)
5'3"	109 (105-113)	116 (110-122)	126 (118-134)
5'4"	112 (108-116)	120 (113-126)	130 (121-138)
5'5"	115 (111-119)	123 (116-130)	134 (125-142)
5'6"	119 (114-123)	128 (120-135)	138 (129-146)
5'7"	123 (118-127)	132 (124-139)	142 (133-150)
5'8"	127 (122-131)	136 (128-143)	146 (137-154)
5'9"	131 (126-135)	140 (132-147)	150 (141-158)
5'10"	135 (130-140)	144 (136-151)	154 (145-163)
5'11"	139 (134-144)	148 (140-155)	159 (149-168)
6'0"	143 (138-148)	152 (144-159)	163 (153-173)
6'1"	—	—	—
6'2"	—	—	—
6'3"	—	—	—
6'4"	—	—	—

The numbers in parentheses are reproduced with permission from the Metropolitan Life Insurance Company's Desirable Weight Table

So now that you have decided to lose weight, follow the six steps to understanding *The California Diet*.

1. How To Find Your Maintenance Calorie Intake.

For each person of a certain ideal weight there is a daily calorie intake that will just maintain weight and sustain a sedentary lifestyle. Most people who are significantly overweight are not very active — they don't play much. So for them, this calorie intake (their Maintenance Calorie Intake) is all it takes to keep them fat, and they are probably slowly gaining weight on this amount of food. These maintenance intakes are shown in the following table. Notice that they seem to be quite modest daily intakes; but this is all it takes to keep you fat if you are not very playful! Again, these figures are approximate, because of individual variation.

So, find your Ideal Weight from the previous table, and then read your approximate Maintenance Calorie Intake from the following table (Our man with an ideal weight of 145 pounds has a maintenance level of 2200 calories per day.):

IDEAL WEIGHT	MAINTENANCE CALORIE INTAKE
(Pounds)	(Low to Moderate Activity)
87-100	1400
101-114	1600
115-126	1800
127-139	2000
140-153	2200
154-166	2400
167-179	2600
180-193	2800

2. Follow the Eat and Play Plan That Is Right for You.

First find your correct plan (these are located in Part IV, pages 195-202) by looking for your Maintenance Calorie Intake. We will go through the plan, using our man who has an ideal weight of 145 pounds, but actually weighs 175 pounds, and wishes to lose 30 pounds. His entry level is 2200 calories. The plan covers a one-year period divided into months. The top part of the plan looks like this:

THE CALIFORNIA DIET EAT AND PLAY PLANS

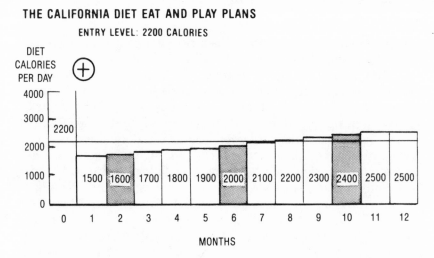

This part of the plan is marked with a⊕to show that calories are being put into the system each month as food. The entry level of 2200 calories drops to 1500 for the first month of the plan. The calorie level then increases by 100 calories per day each month until the original maintenance level is reached by month eight. The level then increases by 100 calories per month to month 11, and remains at 2500 calories per day for month 12. This is 300 calories per day *above* the entry level. The black bars at 1600, 2000 and 2400 calories per day indicate a new Calorie Plan. The total food intake in one year for this plan is approximately 735,000 calories!

Below the calorie intake plan is the Play Plan, which looks like this:

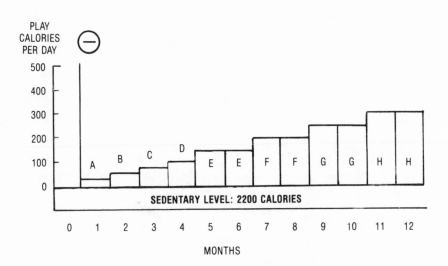

This chart shows the number of calories per day that our man will expend each month on *extra* play. All of these figures are in addition to the basic 2200 calorie maintenance level needed for a sedentary existence. In the first month, 25 calories per day of *extra* play is enjoyed, as Play Plan A. Level A activity is tied (linked, rivetted, bonded, welded, lashed, chained and manacled) to the 1500 Calorie Plan at the 2200 calorie entry level. The 1500 Calorie Plan and Play Plan A go together like bacon and eggs and *must not be separated.* Next month it's Play Plan B, inseparably linked to a 1600 Calorie Plan, and so on to the end of the year, as indicated, until Play Plan H (300 calories per day) goes with the 2500 Calorie Plan. This chart is marked ⊖ to signify that these are calories leaving the system during play (together with the 2200 basic calories). At the end of the year, the calorie expenditure is 300 calories above the sedentary entry level, exactly balancing the 300 extra calories in the 2500 calorie diet plan of month 12. The total calorie expenditure in one year is about 835,000 calories!

The next lower part of the plan looks like this:

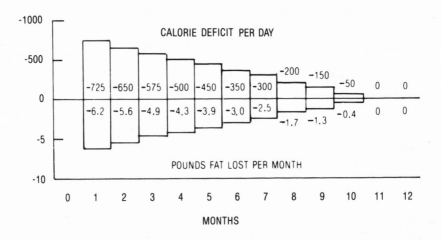

The upper part of the chart shows for each month the calorie deficit per day. This is simply the difference between calories added from the diet and calories subtracted by the basic need (2200) plus the Play Plan. Thus for month one:

1500 calories in *minus* 2225 calories out = − 725 calories per day

This is energy that *must* come from body stores, particularly from fat. Notice that the plan results in steadily decreasing deficits as the year proceeds. For the last two months the equation is:

2500 calories in *minus* 2500 calories out = 0 calories per day

At this point (in all plans) the body is in balance, neither gaining nor losing calories (or fat). This is the condition we need to reach, one of equilibrium. Weight-loss plans should end in this way, as *The California Diet* does.

The lower part of this section of the plan shows for each month the effect of all this on your body fat. One pound of fat contains (and is made from) *about* 3500 calories. So a loss of 725 calories per day for the first month is 21,750 calories. Divided by 3500, this translates into a body fat loss of about 6.2 pounds, as shown.

Body fat declines each month until, in months 11 and 12, the steady state is reached, no fat is lost or gained, and the weight-loss plan ends where it should end, in a state of equilibrium.

Finally, at the bottom of each plan there is a boxed summary of the outcome of the year's plan. It looks like this:

Calorie deficit one year — 118,500 Calories

Fat loss one year — 34 Pounds

Weight loss one year — 30 Pounds

The calorie deficit for one year is the total shortage of energy, energy provided by food, in relation to the expenditure in basic living plus play. The deficit comes to a grand total of 118,500 calories *in the hole*. Of course, this loss has to come from somewhere, and the body takes it from fat supplies. So divide 118,500 by 3500 (one pound of fat in calories) and we get about 34 pounds lost. This is our man's weight loss at the end of the year, then? Well, not exactly, because all that play has added some muscle. He looks much better because the four pounds of muscle he has gained helps to tighten up his body where fat has been lost. His net weight loss is 30 pounds, exactly his target weight loss. This would be a very satisfactory result for him, of course. It is unlikely that you will come out *exactly* at the weight loss the plan indicates; but if carefully followed, with conscientious coupling of the appropriate Play Plan with the calorie plan, you should come within a few pounds of the stated weight loss.

The entire plan for our representative man looks like this:

THE CALIFORNIA DIET EAT AND PLAY PLANS
ENTRY LEVEL: 2200 CALORIES

2200

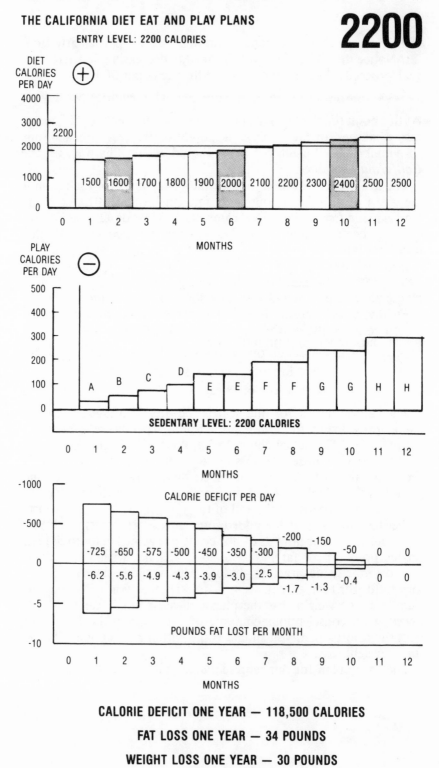

CALORIE DEFICIT ONE YEAR — 118,500 CALORIES

FAT LOSS ONE YEAR — 34 POUNDS

WEIGHT LOSS ONE YEAR — 30 POUNDS

Get familiar with your plan — you will live with it for a year. Remember, if your weight loss is slower than the plan shows (and you have conscientiously linked the Calorie Plan with the Play Plan for two months), switch to the next lower Eat and Play Plan. Our man would switch to the 2000 Calorie Plan. This means that calorie intake will be further reduced.

Take it a month at a time and remember, it is not long until you get to play more and eat more!

Don't worry that your weight loss gradually slows: it's supposed to! You can't go on losing forever! Your plan will bring you to a smooth landing at the end of the year at your new weight — fit, eating more and better able to control your weight in the future.

3. How to Use the Calorie Plans

The Calorie Plans, to help you obtain the correct calorie intake at all stages of your plan, are located in Part IV, pages 203-230. The plans are for these daily major calorie levels: 1200, 1600, 2000, 2400, 2800. Each plan is for seven days, and gives menus for breakfast, lunch and dinner, and (in most plans) snacks.

Day 1 of the 1200 Calorie Plan looks like this:

1200 CALORIE PLAN

SAMPLE MENUS — BASED ON EXCHANGE LISTS

DAY 1	
BREAKFAST	Orange juice, ½ cup (D); Non-fat milk, 1 cup (Al); whole grain cereal, cooked, ½ cup (E) with 2 tablespoons raisins (D) and 7 almonds (H)
LUNCH	Non-fat milk, 1 cup (Al); Sandwich: whole grain bread, 2 slices (E), skim milk cheese, 2 ounces (F1); Salad: spinach, 1 cup (B) with ½ tablespoon dressing (H); Cantaloupe, ¼ (6 inches) (D)
DINNER	Chinese beef with vegetables® , 1 serving; Rice, cooked, ½ cup (E); Lettuce salad, 1 cup (B) with 2 tablespoons low-calorie dressing® (LCD)

There are several things to notice. Recipes for some dishes are given (in Part IV, pages 251-277) where marked (e.g., Chinese Beef with Vegetables®). Following each item in the menu (except the recipes) is a capitalized letter or a letter with a number, in parentheses:

Orange Juice, ½ cup (D)

The letter (D) refers you to the Exchange Lists (located in Part IV, pages 231-250).This enables you to exchange any item on the menu for an equivalent item (equivalent in calorie and nutrient content), as described in the next section.

At the back of each Calorie Plan is a Daily Food Allowance and a Typical Meal Pattern for that plan. The Daily Food Allowance for the 1200 Calorie Plan looks like this:

1200 CALORIE PLAN

DAILY FOOD ALLOWANCE

FOOD GROUP	NUMBER OF SERVINGS	CHOOSE FROM LIST
Milk	2	A1
Vegetables	2-4	B
Fruits	3	D
Bread	4	E
Protein Foods		
Animal	5	F1
Vegetable	1	G1, 2
Fats	3	H
Free Foods	As Desired (AD)	I

This allows you to make up your own calorie plans if you prefer, using the foods given in the Exchange Lists.

The Typical Meal Pattern for 1200 calories looks like this:

TYPICAL MEAL PATTERN

BREAKFAST
1 Serving Milk (A1)
2 Servings Fruit (D)
1 Serving Bread (E)
1 Serving Fat (H)

LUNCH
1 Servings Milk (A1)
At least 1 Serving Vegetable (B)
1 Serving Fruit (D)
2 Servings Bread (E)
2 Servings Animal Protein (F1)
1 Serving Vegetable Protein (G1, 2) (or at dinner)
1 Serving Fat (H)

DINNER
At least 1 Serving Vegetable (B)
1 Serving Bread (E)
3 Servings Animal Protein (F1)
1 Serving Vegetable Protein (G1, 2) (or at lunch)
1 Serving Fat (H)

SNACK
AD Free Foods (I)

This suggests a pattern for distributing the foods from the various food groups throughout the day, if you are making up your own calorie plans.

There is one other major point. Your Eat and Play Plan will show daily calorie levels *between* the major calorie plan levels: 1200, 1600, 2000, 2400, 2800. When you are in a month between these major levels, you must supplement the next lower Calorie Plan. For instance, our representative man, with his 2200 calorie Eat and Play Plan, starts out in his first month with 1500 calories per day. So he must add 300 calories per day to the next lower 1200 Calorie Plan to bring it up to 1500 calories. He does this by choosing foods he likes from Exchange Lists B, C, D or E (vegetables, fruits and breads, the high-carbohydrate foods). If you are on a 2600 calorie month, follow the major 2400 Calorie Plan and choose another 200 calories per day from the Exchange Lists. When your plan advances to the next *major* calorie level, transfer to that plan, without supplementing. So, our man supplements the 1200 Calorie Plan to get 1500 calories for his first month; but the next month he moves to a completely new 1600 Calorie Plan (page 208). The following month he supplements the 1600 Calorie Plan by 100 calories (from the Exchange Lists) and so has a 1700 Calorie Plan for that month. In this way, calorie levels are gradually built back up as play level increases, and there is something more to look forward to as each month goes by.

You may not like some items in your Calorie Plan. *Exchange* them for equivalent items, using the Exchange Lists. You will notice that the calorie plans do not contain sweet desserts (e.g., cake, ice cream) or alcoholic drinks. These are not forbidden. You can read more about the pros and cons of sugar and alcohol as dietary components later in the book. If you want to include these items in your plans, within the total calorie allowance you are following, do so by selecting items from Exchange List J. This will allow you to include sweet desserts and/or alcoholic drinks in your plan whenever you are supplementing a basic Calorie Plan. You may think of these additions as rewards or treats to celebrate advancing to a new, higher calorie level and, of course, advancing to a new, higher play level. For instance, if you are advancing from 2200 calories to 2300 calories, you might select one four-ounce glass of white wine, *or* ⅓ cup of ice cream (from Exchange List J) as your way of adding 100 calories per day to the 2200 calorie plan, and as your reward.

What's contained in your Calorie Plan meals? Approximately the stated number of calories, of course. But in *The California Diet* care has also been taken to provide all the important nutrients you will need. Many diet plans do not do this (some are totally inadequate in many respects). Your present diet may be inadequate in some ways. The plans given here will provide ample amounts of nutrients (protein, vitamins, minerals) and other components (e.g., fiber) to maintain good health, and are low in items that should be low (salt, cholesterol, saturated fat). More about this in Part III.

At the end of each Calorie Plan is the Nutritional Content. For the 1200 Calorie Plan it looks like this:

NUTRITIONAL CONTENT

(AVERAGE DAILY INTAKE OVER SEVEN DAYS OF PLAN)

CALORIES	1232
PROTEIN (grams)	87
TOTAL FAT (grams)	27
TOTAL CARBOHYDRATES (grams)	160
% PROTEIN CALORIES	28
% FAT CALORIES	20
% CARBOHYDRATE CALORIES	52
POLYUNSATURATED/SATURATED FAT (P/S) RATIO	1.08
REFINED SUGAR (grams)	1
NATURAL SIMPLE SUGARS (grams)	75
STARCH (grams)	77
CHOLESTEROL (milligrams)	151
CALCIUM (milligrams)	1007
PHOSPHORUS (milligrams)	1472
MAGNESIUM (milligrams)	352
IRON (milligrams)	17
ZINC (milligrams)	13
VITAMIN A (International units)	12,203
THIAMINE (milligrams)	1.3
RIBOFLAVIN (milligrams)	2.2
NIACIN (milligrams)	20
VITAMIN C (milligrams)	180
VITAMIN B_6 (milligrams)	2.1
FOLACIN (micrograms)	285

This gives the calculated average content of nutrients for the 1200 Calorie Plan over the entire seven days. You will see calories, protein, fat and carbohydrate content, vitamins, minerals, sugar, cholesterol, saturated and polyunsaturated fat content — and no alcohol. As mentioned earlier, you can add alcohol to *supplement* the major calorie plans (1200, 1600, 2000, 2400, 2800 calories).

4. How to Use the Exchange Lists.

These diets are based on the exchange principle. After all, not everyone wants to eat the same thing, and we all like a change. So exchange! The Exchange Lists allow you to do this freely, while still staying within your calorie plan, and still getting balanced, nutritious meals. The Exchange Lists (in Part IV, pages 231-250) are as follows:

A   Milk Exchange

B/C Vegetable Exchange
    B — Low calories
    C — 50 calories per ½ cup

D   Fruit Exchange

E   Bread Exchange

F/G Protein Exchange

Animal Products:

    F1 — Lean Meat
    F2 — Medium Fat
    F3 — High Fat

Vegetable Products:

    G1 — Low Fat
    G2 — Medium Fat
    G3 — High Fat

H   Fat Exchange

I   Free Foods
(no calories)

J   Additional List
(includes alcohol and desserts)

The Milk Exchange looks like this:

A. MILK EXCHANGE

A1. Non-Fat	**Serving Size**	**Grams**
(Each serving = 80 calories)		
Skim milk	1 cup	240
Powdered (non-fat, dry)	¼ cup	35
Buttermilk made from skim milk	1 cup	240
Canned, evaporated-skim milk	½ cup	120
Yogurt made from skim milk (plain)	1 cup	240
A2. Low-Fat		
(Each serving = 120 calories)		
Low-fat milk (2% fat)	1 cup	240
Yogurt made from 2% fat milk)	1 cup	240
A3. Whole Milk		
(Each serving = 160 calories)		
Whole milk	1 cup	240
Canned, evaporated whole milk	½ cup	120
Powdered milk (whole, dry)	¼ cup	35
Buttermilk made from whole milk	1 cup	240
Yogurt made from whole milk (plain)	1 cup	240

This list shows the kinds and amounts of milk or milk products to use for one Milk Exchange. Adults as well as children need the nutrients found in milk, particularly calcium and riboflavin. It is also a good source of protein, phosphorus, vitamins A, B$_{12}$, and, if fortified, vitamin D.

If you are unable to eat milk products, it is important to substitute other foods that are rich in calcium such as blackstrap molasses, sunflower and sesame seeds, bok choy, kale, mustard greens, broccoli, asparagus, okra, tofu, dandelion greens, dry beans, soy beans, cabbage, rutabagas, turnips, carrots, dates, figs, oranges and whole wheat bread. Calcium is important for the health of bones, teeth and muscles.

Each Exchange List states clearly the calorie content of each item. You need to know this to be able to supplement in units of approximately 100 calories per day as you go through your California Diet Eat and Play Plans. For instance, each non-fat milk exchange is approximately 80 calories. Milk exchanges fall into one of three categories, depending on fat content. So you might exchange two A1 items (one cup of skim milk for one cup of plain yogurt made from skim milk) or two A3 items (½ cup of canned, evaporated whole milk for one cup of buttermilk made from whole milk). You will soon get a feel for the use of the exchange system by looking through the Exchange Lists on pages 231-250. Some useful comments and nutritional significance of the foods are given for each list.

Remember:

• Exchange symbol for symbol (e.g., F2 for F2; not, for example, F1 for F2) in the Calorie Plans.

• Look for the calorie contents of items when supplementing basic Calorie Plans.

• The exchanges are approximate, not exact.

5. How To Use the Recipes

In Part IV, you will find the recipes that are marked in the Calorie Plans like this: ® . They are arranged in alphabetical order so you can more easily find them. The first recipe looks like this:

APPLE AND ENDIVE SALAD

2 tablespoons lemon juice
4 small apples, cored, cut into ¼ inch slices
½ cup celery, diced
4 small endives, cored, cut into 2-inch strips*
2 tablespoons oil
12 whole broken walnuts
1 tablespoon minced mint or parsley leaves

Drizzle lemon juice over sliced apples; toss well. Mix in celery, endives, and oil. Just before serving, stir in walnuts. Garnish with mint or parsley. Serves 4.

Each serving=180 Calories
                1 Vegetable Exchange (B)
                1 Fruit Exchange (D)
                3 Fat Exchanges (H)
*If not available, 2 cups torn lettuce may be substituted
Time: 15 minutes

Most recipes make several servings. Only one serving is used in the calorie plans. At the bottom of each recipe you will find the approximate calorie content per serving, and also the type and number of food exchanges contained in one serving. This recipe makes 4 servings. Each serving contains 180 calories, and one vegetable exchange (B), one fruit exchange (D) and three fat exchanges (H).

6. How to Use the Play Plans.

The Play Plans are a vital part of your total California Diet and Exercise Program. Each day, choose from the activities listed on the Play Plan you are following for a given month. Do not jump ahead on Play Plans; the system is designed so that you progress very gradually from a sedentary to a fit state, without sudden increases. In this way you will avoid injuries (see Part II). Play Plans run from A to J (25 to 500 play calories per day) and are located in Part IV, pages 272-277.

The first Play Plan (A) looks like this:

PLAY PLAN A
(25 calories per day)

(25)

Choose *one* playful act *each day* from the accompanying list. These are *extra* play calories to *add* to your usual routine:
  Walk a quarter-mile (3 blocks)
  Cycle a mile, slowly
  Swim for 3 minutes
  Dance (aerobic) for 5 minutes
  Clean windows for 6 minutes
  Rake leaves for 6 minutes
  Scrub floors for 6 minutes
Feel free to try different activities on different days.

PLAYFUL HINTS . . .
• Get off to a good start — don't overdo!
• Find a playful friend!
• Don't forget — keep your play record.
• Yes — it's easy to start with, but there's lots more fun to come!

Read Part II of this book for further suggestions and hints to make the Play Plan fun — and effective! This is the crucial part of your *California Diet*. Think of the Play Plans as all part of the Calorie Plans. The Play Plans make the calorie plans work!

4. Is There Life
After Weight Loss?

To conclude Part I, I'll assume that you have been persuaded by the various arguments of the earlier chapters, have adopted *The California Diet*, and have successfully lost weight over a period of one year, becoming a playful person in the process. Let's look at that great number of person-years that lie ahead.

HEALTH AND VITALITY THROUGH THE LIFE SPAN

There is a good deal of talk these days about the "aging American population." This phenomenon shows up in various areas of our national activities. Social Security has to adapt to the probability that the ratio of older, retired people taking money out of the system compared to younger working people putting money into the system, will slowly increase. The need for housing is changing from large homes with lots of bedrooms for the children to smaller homes for two or three people. The demand for specialist physicians will probably change, with less call for pediatricians and more for gerontologists.

This changing situation, being experienced in many developed countries, has come about because people are living longer on average. There are two things to consider: This does not mean that there will be many more *extremely* old people (nineties and beyond) in the population, and it does not *necessarily* mean that the population will enjoy itself more. Drs. James Fries and Lawrence Crapo, of Stanford University Medical School, have looked carefully at the past, present and future of aging in America, and have reflected on the consequences for the nation's vitality. The accompanying diagram is very revealing as we scan the horizon to see what lies ahead.

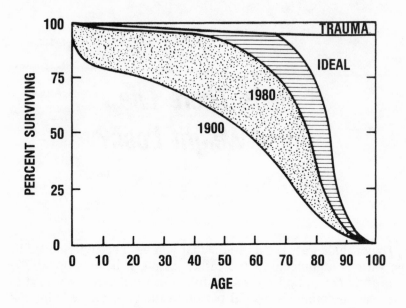

The Ideal Survival Curve (from James F. Fries and Lawrence M. Crapo, *Vitality and Aging,* W.H. Freeman and Company, San Francisco, 1981).

The first curve shows the way in which our grandparents or great grandparents and their families left this earthly life in 1900. For each hundred babies born, there was a high infant mortality, reducing the 100 to 90 after only one year. By the end of 20 years, only 75 remained, as the terrible diseases of those days — tuberculosis, pneumonia, diphtheria, typhoid and measles took their yearly toll of young people. The major infectious diseases continued to remove middle-aged adults from the surviving population, until chronic diseases such as cancer and heart disease took over for those surviving to 60 and beyond. Now look at the curve for 1980; it is very different. Infant mortality is greatly reduced, and through the age of about 45 it is rather uncommon to die of any cause other than trauma (auto accidents, homicide, suicide). Beyond age 45, the great chronic diseases, particularly heart disease, stroke and cancers, take their toll and prevent large numbers of middle-aged to elderly people from completing their maximum biological life span, which appears to be 85 to 95 for the vast majority of people. Finally, you will see a curve marked "Ideal." This represents the "best" experience that we can expect, as a population, short of remarkable and presently unlikely scientific breakthroughs that push our "normal" life span into the hundreds. In these ideal circumstances, virtually no individual would be removed from the population before age 70. Even trauma, which is shown on the diagram taking its toll all across the life span, might be considerably reduced by attention to vehicular safety and handgun control, both of which are well within our power to influence.

The area on the diagram between the line marked "1900" and the line marked "Ideal" gives a visual impression of the *maximum* extension of lives that medical science and attention to public health could achieve, as viewed in 1900. The speckled area between "1900" and "1980" shows the spectacular gains that have been made already, through better housing and sanitation, cleaner food, less crowding, antibiotics, vaccines and improved nutrition, among many other twentieth century wonders. This is what our health dollar has bought us: more life for young people, children, teenagers, young adults, and for middle-aged adults. The very oldest people in our population are not living longer, and are not likely to, even under ideal circumstances. It is nothing short of astonishing that some 80 percent of the vast task of life-salvage that confronted the public health establishment in 1900 has already been achieved by the 1980s. Only 20 percent more remains to be achieved, and you can see from the diagram that this last effort, via smoking prevention, blood pressure control and some surgical techniques, for example, is going to give extra years of life predominantly to people who have *already* lived for 60, 70 and 80 years.

The diagram shows us what has happened to life expectancies in the United States, and how the changes in need for housing, retirement benefits and physician care have come about. The American male, with a current life expectancy at birth of 70 years, and the female, with 78 years, can only be described on the basis of historical experience, as "long-lived." As Fries and Crapo put it: "Clearly, the medical and social task of eliminating premature death . . . is largely accomplished."

The achievements of the past 80 years, the elimination of all those sad, early deaths of sons and daughters, the banishment of the specters of polio and syphilis, all of this has been magnificent. But what does it have to do with *The California Diet*?

Everything we have just considered relates particularly to how long people live — and much less to the quality of their lives. It is precisely because we are all destined to live longer from now on that we particularly need to pay attention to the quality of life in the fifties, sixties and seventies. We need to stretch our ideas of the "useful," "productive," "attractive" and "enjoyable" years of our lives to incorporate these decades, or we will rapidly have a huge, unproductive, unhappy, "left out" segment of the population on our hands. Now is the time for people in their forties and fifties to plan *not* for retirement, but for an influential, important, productive, enjoyable 20 years — the sixties and seventies.

Now, the sixties and seventies may not sound very productive and enjoyable to younger people today. Why? Because in the younger mind — yours, perhaps — are images of 60- and 70-year-old relatives and friends. Uncle Fred, in and out of hospital with his heart problem and emphysema; hardly enjoying life in his sixties, retired, but seldom able to get out into his garden. And Auntie Flo, very overweight, arthritic, chained to the television set, inactive and dependent in her early seventies. And this is what medical progress has given us, the gift of extended life? Clearly, the images, and the reality, must be changed for social, economic and humanitarian reasons.

There are, after all, many 70-year-olds with exacting, influential positions in society — senators, businessmen, teachers — and many with good lungs and hearts, and slim figures. Did you know that the pole vault record for 66-year-old men is 11 feet 10 inches (a long way to come down!) and the age 65 marathon (26 miles 385 yards) record for women is less than four hours? In other words, many older people are capable of performances in many of life's endeavors that are the envy of much younger people. This means that the years from 50 to 80 do not have to be afflicted with decreasing mobility and physical performance, and with increasing dependence and medical expense. The caricature we see of the older person features wheelchairs and sedentariness and often obesity; but this need not be so and, as the future descends upon us, must not be so.

The physical condition we exhibit in later years depends to a considerable extent on the way we live our earlier years. There is evidence, for instance, that debilitating heart conditions result from smoking, an unfavorable blood cholesterol pattern, high blood pressure, poor diet and being overweight; that most lung diseases afflicting older people are cigarette-related; that regular exercise leads to a good body weight, improved cholesterol pattern and reduced inclination to smoke. People in their thirties and forties today who choose a healthy lifestyle are going to be the people tomorrow who enjoy their sixties and seventies. *The California Diet* is designed to do much more than reduce your weight over a few months and then abandon you. It leads you to a lifestyle that is more active, enables you to eat more and, most importantly, to eat more healthily. It also (as your activity increases) weans you from smoking, while gradually reducing your body fat and toning your muscles. The entire program contains the most modern features required to *lower* your risk in later years of developing heart disease, lung diseases, some cancers, osteoporosis, obesity and premature immobility.

Gradualness

People who are very fit and slim did not become that way overnight. The 60-year-old who can get out his bicycle and ride 30 miles didn't suddenly jump on a new bicycle after years of inactivity and cover that distance on the first day. The 50-year-old woman who regularly runs in the local 10-kilometer road races started, one day, by jogging one block. All achievement comes gradually, and the more gadually it comes the more permanently it stays. That is why *The California Diet* is gradual. The moderate reduction of calories you experience in the first month of your plan is *gradually* increased, month by month. The increase is not large: The second month you will be adding 100 or 50 or even zero calories to your daily menu, but the improvement is *progressive*. There is something to look forward to all the time. As we all know, the months fly by, and before you know it you are at month eight and back to about the calorie level you were on before you started the program. And all the time your play level is gradually, almost imperceptibly picking up. The first month you simply walk three blocks or rake leaves for six minutes! Some sort of exercise program this is! But don't hurry it. You must get into the habit of playing gradually. If the play is ridiculously easy the first month, it's ridiculously easy to fit it in, not to forget it. And if you are really out of shape, your muscles and tendons are weak and yet carrying an overweight you, they need time very gradually to get the message: The lazy, playless days are over! Shape up! And before you know it you are into your second month and exploring six street blocks each day, or aerobic dancing for 10 minutes. The gradual increase in play will make you feel due for a reward, and the natural reward, what your body really wants, is food. So you will feel appropriately self-righteous each month when your calorie plan takes a jump, because you have earned it, each day of the previous month. But remember, the key to successful play, eating and weight loss is *gradualness*.

Staying With It

If the weight (I should say fat) you have lost on a diet begins to return (and this is the case for the majority of dieters) you can look at two sides of the problem: You are beginning to eat too much; or you are not playing enough. Or you may be a bit off in both directions. Most diet programs, anticipating the weight regain problem, will concentrate on eating habits. Typical instructions might include:
- Serve only small portions of food
- Keep high-calorie items out of sight
- Pause between each bite
- Take smaller bites

- Drink water between each bite
- Consciously eat very s-l-o-w-l-y.

You can immediately see all of these instructions as tricks to keep food out of your body. They may have some place, especially for the lifelong compulsive overeater who needs to lose a very large amount of fat; but this program is not for him. As I have already emphasized, the moderately overweight person who has become the victim of creeping inactivity over the last 20 to 30 years is *not eating too much.* His problem is grossly inadequate physical activity. Therefore, for this person, prescribing a set of behavioral devices designed to further reduce his already inadequate food intake is hardly the proper way to proceed: it is curing a disease that doesn't exist. This does bring up the thought that many weight-loss programs, concentrating on the "eat less" approach as a task of behavioral re-education, were probably devised in the rather unusual setting of a hospital weight-loss clinic specializing in a relatively small minority of clients with a specific eating disorder: eating considerably too much! My audience, a vast one, has different problems: a rather severe inactivity problem coupled with a mild case of the opposite type of eating disorder: eating too little! The solution, then, is to promote increased activity in as pleasant and playful a way as possible. This is where the emphasis must be — where the greatest problem is. At the same time, surplus fat has *very slowly* accumulated on your body over the years, and you want to remove it. So the combination of mild, *temporary* dieting and increasing exercise is indicated. But remember that the underlying fault is the inactivity, not the eating pattern. So I do not want you to practice taking micro-bites or hiding food or meditating between mouthfuls.

If you have successfully lost weight on *The California Diet* but are now regaining it, think "play." This is what has gone wrong. Concentrate on the middle section of this book and get back to being playful. Has something happened that has reduced your play? Is it a cold winter, so you are getting out less? Pursue indoor activities: aerobic dancing, disco dancing, swimming indoors. Invest in some warmer sports clothes to tempt you outdoors. Try to exercise during midday, when it's warmer. Has a friend left town, so you have nobody to nudge you to play? The world is full of friends — find another one and *you* nudge him!

If your recent weight gain is accompanied with generally "not feeling so lively," you can be sure (in the absence of real illness) that your play level is slipping. It is a curious and sad consequence of our modern super-mechanized, computerized, step-saving lives that we can underexercise ourselves *en masse* into a morbid state, a state we do not even recognize, of overweight, undereating and generally "not feeling good." And the solution to that, dear friends, is not "smaller bites."

Going Round Again

Some readers who are at the higher end of the "moderately overweight" spectrum may go through the one-year *California Diet* and come out 30 pounds lighter, and fitter. But if you could reasonably afford to lose 60 pounds at the start of the program, you might like to take off another 30. How do the plans accommodate this? You can always go back again to the beginning of your plan. For instance, if you were on the 2200 Calorie Plan, you are now (at the end of the year) on 2500 calories, and burning an extra 300 calories on Play Plan H. *Don't reduce your play level!* That is the last thing you want to do in order to lose more weight. Keep your exercise level the same, and go back to the calorie plan of month one, 1500 calories. You now have a calorie deficit of 1000 calories per day, and will lose weight rapidly. Each month you increase your calorie intake according to the plan, and your rate of weight loss will gradually decrease. If you achieve your goal of losing another 30 pounds before the year is out, you can return to the 2500 calorie level, which is balancing your activity level, and then your new, lower weight should be just maintained.

A better, alternative way to lose another 30 pounds on the 2200 Calorie Plan is to return to an intermediate calorie level, say 1800 calories per day, while maintaining your 300 calorie Play Plan H level. You will start to lose weight. Each month increase your diet calories by 100. After four months go to Play Plan I (400 calories per day) and after eight months go to Play Plan J (500 calories per day). Adjust your diet over the last two months of the year to 2700 calories, so that your calorie expenditure (2200 entry, plus 500 play calories) just balances your food intake. By the end of this second year you should be very fit, walking five miles each day, for instance, about 60 pounds lighter than you were and regularly eating a handsome 2700 calories each day.

Anyone who has lived with the Eat and Play Plans for a year will be able easily to tailor them to particular needs. More than anything, the one-year experience should teach the supreme importance of our play levels in controlling weight. In fact, at the higher play levels (Plans I and J) it is typical that participants don't need to watch *how much* they eat anymore. This is the condition of the middle-aged jogger who runs several miles every day, eats as much as his appetite dictates and remains slim. This is the way we are intended to be — not constantly calorie counting.

Notice that I say "as much" as his appetite dictates, not

"whatever his appetite dictates." The appetite in an active, playful person is a reliable guide to proper calorie intake, but is not very reliable when it comes to the type or quality of food. As we shall see in Part III of this book, the quality of our diet is also of great importance for our future health and well-being. But after a year on your plan you should be quite familiar with the types and combinations of foods that give you a relatively low-fat, low-cholesterol, low-salt diet that is rich in minerals, vitamins and fiber, while also being attractive and appetizing.

In summary, anyone who has successfully lost weight by following *The California Diet* for one year should have no problem "going round again" for additional weight loss. Maintenance, and increase of your play level is the key to success. And be sure to keep up a *healthy* diet to safeguard your future vitality.

Is There Life After Weight Loss?

For most of my readers there is life after weight loss: lots and lots of it. I have tried to point out that the gift of life, the extra years to live, is being given more and more to Americans who are already middle-aged. We asked for it, we got it, let's enjoy it!

A weight-loss program should consider not only how to remove weight this month, but how to keep it off in 30 years time; it should consider not how to deceive the body into eating less now, but how to repair the most common underlying fault responsible for moderate obesity: inactivity.

With vast numbers of Americans headed toward an extended life span, it is increasingly important that they undertake the journey well equipped for the years to come. Our vocabulary needs extending, our understanding of words, modifying. "Old age" has a terrifying ring about it. We have to change all that now — it's out of date. Because that is what medical science is about to award us with — "old age." Perhaps, like obsolete words that have acquired unpleasant ethnic or sexual overtones, "old age" and its synonyms should be discarded. How about "play time" or "opportunity time"? And "re-entry" instead of "retirement"?

And medical science must be pressed much harder to improve our *enjoyment* of those extra years, not simply to make them tolerable. The huge, expensive machine of medical care and research has to be redirected. Its success in prolonging life has been spectacular. Now we must wind it up again and set it to the task of making our full life span productive and enjoyable. We have a tremendous amount to find out; we are like the physicians of 1900, unable to imagine a world with penicillin and polio vaccine; without smallpox and syphilis. The myriad, haunting overtones that once surrounded "childbirth" have now gone, replaced by the largely joyful event we know today. "Old age" is next for the treatment.

It would be verging on the immodest to suggest that this program can help in this huge task. But *The California Diet* does contain several elements that most experts would agree predict a smooth passage into older age: an active life, a healthy diet and easily maintained slimness.

PART TWO: LEARNING TO PLAY AGAIN

5. Exercise as Play, Not Work

VOICES FROM OUR EVOLUTIONARY PAST

Changes in all aspects of our lives have gone on at breakneck speed in the past 80 years. We have seen the effect of public health advances, in particular the shift in the makeup of our population toward a greater proportion of older citizens. The way in which we occupy our days, whether working days or leisure days, has also changed incredibly fast. Not long ago the Want Ads page in the newspaper offered a good number of quite active jobs: digging ditches, carrying heavy loads or walking much of the day. Most of these jobs have gone, victims of machines. A machine can dig a better ditch, faster. A machine can harvest tomatoes or trim hedges. Indeed, scientists who study the influence on health of vigorous activity compared to sedentary occupations, have had to turn to people engaged in vigorous *leisure time* activities, since there are so few large groups of people now regularly performing truly vigorous occupational work. A good example is the longshoreman — once a lifter, a carrier and a shoveler, now an operator of a moving belt or a forklift truck. Unemployment has been climbing in the United States and other developed countries in recent years, partly because of a worldwide recession, but also because of the steady elimination of many jobs that required much muscle but little training. In fact, even at the height of the recent recession, there are many jobs available, if you can program computers or run an office: *not*, notice, if you can walk or carry or saw wood all day.

If we look at the many tasks done by homemakers, or by the gainfully employed on their weekends and days off, we see further enormous changes. So many machines now do things we used to do with muscle, whether it's the power lawn mower or the electric hedge clipper, the electric floor scrubber or the telephone, "to let your fingers do the walking." Opportunities to use muscles evaporate at an alarming rate; some are major opportunities like sawing wood (replaced by the chain saw), while others are tiny ones like washing dishes (replaced by the automatic dishwasher). But they all add up.

The automobile, of course, has had a vast influence on our society, much of it for the good. The bad consequences are clear, too: road accidents, pollution, energy dependence. If you read Chapter 8, you will find a long catalog of the beneficial effects of exercise. It is unlikely that Henry Ford had any inkling of the health ramifications of his invention, as America rapidly chose to ride, rather than walk. This does make us pause to wonder what unforeseen health consequences may result in 20 years time from the current massive new trends, such as widespread acceptance of home computers. Increased sedentariness, as we press buttons rather than actually get up and visit the bank, for example, seems likely to be one. Another relatively recent event with possible health consequences is the widespread use of the motor scooter. To the extent that use of these motorized bicycles replaces use of a larger, four-wheeled motorized vehicle, I suppose this is all to the good. But how often is the walk to work, or the stroll down to the store, now replaced by the easier trip on the motor scooter?

In most areas it seems probable that the sedentary plague can only spread. The Energy Crisis promised to restore walking to favor, but motor scooters and alternative energy sources seem more popular solutions for many. The silicon chip and its successors are also set to shape the future. Sitting in front of the computer screen seems likely to be a major part of almost everyone's job before long; and how many generations will pass before small boys abandon video games for the old excitement of real-life games in the open air?

We get a rather gloomy impression from all this. Exercise is good for us, yet opportunities to do it at work or in the home seem to be disappearing at an alarming rate. But, you will be saying, "What about the Great American Exercise Explosion? All those joggers in the parks? All those new racquetball courts?" And, of course, this has been the great reaction, the huge revolution that has, mercifully, helped to correct a rapidly deteriorating national situation. But note that in spite of this upsurge in *leisure* activity, the American overweight problem has not noticeably improved. And surveys indicate that vast segments of our population get quite inadequate amounts of regular exercise. My impression is that the relatively recent, laudable and highly visible exercise habits of, perhaps, 25 percent of the population have just managed to offset the further inroads of sedentariness to which the *entire* population is exposed when not consciously choosing to "exercise." In other words, I believe there is no reason for complacency because:

• Our non-leisure "work" activities are becoming more and more sedentary.

• While the leisure-time exercise explosion is highly visible, it is still practiced by a minority of the population; vast numbers of people, those in most need of increased activity, get virtually none.

The numbers and types of Americans who are exercising regularly are very difficult to pin down precisely, and they keep changing. Definitions are very critical. Is the owner of a pair of running shoes a runner? Not necessarily, these days. Is the owner of a bicycle a cyclist? Is a person who took a dip in the pool six times during the hot summer a swimmer? Is a person who runs three miles a week a runner? If 60 million Americans are "swimmers" and 44 million are "cyclists," do we have 104 million regular swimmers and cyclists? Certainly not, since many exercisers do both sports, and many are not "regular." But by all the yardsticks, participation in the major sports — swimming, bicycling, running and jogging, hiking, basketball, softball, tennis, volleyball and roller-skating — has increased greatly in the past 15 years. Yet by the most liberal estimate, only one in three adults even now is regularly obtaining adequate exercise, leaving two in three, or some 120 million, with the serious health disadvantage of inactivity. When we look at subsets of the population, the situation is often much worse. For example, probably less than 10 percent of older women take adequate exercise. You will not be surprised to learn that most of the moderately overweight people in America — my audience — are in the sedentary two-thirds majority.

What got into the minority of men and women who adopted regular exercise? They certainly weren't doing it in 1962, when I arrived in California and was almost arrested when running around the local park at night, in the rain. The tennis courts were empty, and bike paths unheard of. Of course, the growing enthusiasm for exercise was nourished by several outstanding books and magazines, by advertising and by the widely televised Olympic Games. But many thoughtful people in the late 1960s were simply ready for the revolution. Heavy doses of idle, step-saving luxury after World War II, of hot dogs in crowded ball parks, of finned Detroit creations, of more and more television and less and less challenge, with expanding waistlines, prevalent Ugly Americans and soaring heart fatalities, all of this created a large, very receptive revolutionary audience in America. They were receptive to something challenging, health-promoting, admirable and "primeval." The more vigorous sports, especially running, cycling and swimming, had these qualities. And the word spread rapidly. A few tried it, liked it, felt better, looked better, and said so. After a decent period of skepticism, others at the office tried it. A chain reaction had begun, fueled by its own visibility, leading to the relatively widespread popularity of the major non-team sports in America today. This was not a change in American exercise habits resulting from massive government campaigns or from medical edict. There was, in fact, a rather cautious approach to the galloping phenomenon from these quarters. I believe the movement was the result of "modeling" of the activity by a few, followed by the observation that they survived all that dashing about and, in fact, seemed to do well on it. "Have you seen the weight Fred has lost since he took up this jogging? And, God, he *must* be 40!" And as new converts tried the new exercise lifestyle, *they* felt better and told more people, and so on. This is not the mechanism of a fad or a craze. People made an investment, savored the result, and learned something about how to feel well. I believe that the true "fad" was the "inactivity fad" that crept up on America in the guise of the electric golf cart and the televised football game in the 1950s. For perhaps a third of the nation, that fad has passed.

A final thought relates to the "primeval." Our present relatively effortless lifestyle dates back but a few microseconds in the long day of our evolutionary history. It seems that we were intended to be active much of our time. We have our biggest muscles in our legs, for running, walking and jumping. We have a huge world to explore. Days spent at the desk and nights at the television hardly seem to provide the environment we are equipped for. And the need may be more than physical. Perhaps the stockbroker, returning home from sitting down all day, has a real, shallowly covered desire to run out onto his vast forest-covered hunting grounds, to discover what is awaiting him around the next bend, to take some real risks, to run free and unfettered by convention, and to enjoy flexing his physical powers. Well, he can't really do that, but he can change into his running gear and bound out into the street, clad only in his thin uniform, to be blown by the wind, rained upon, pressed physically — things that no other part of his life provides. Perhaps our stockbroker will kick a stone, jump over a park bench, slip in the mud. He can't do this in the office. I call this primeval need "play," following the lead of George Sheehan:

> "Run only if you must. If running is an imperative that comes from inside you and not from your doctor. Otherwise, heed the inner calling to your own Play. Listen if you can to the person you were and can be. Then do what you do best and feel best at. Something you would do for

nothing. Something that gives you security and self-acceptance and a feeling of completion; even moments when you are fused with your universe and your Creator. When you find it, build your life around it."

(Running and Being)

Adventure

The wonderful thing is how so many millions of Americans have incorporated exercise into their otherwise sedentary lives by discovering that it can be an adventure. In this program we should like you to feel the same way. Remember when you were very young, how exciting it was to go out to play? In fact, it was a tragedy if you had to miss it. It seemed this way because you never knew what exciting new play idea someone would come up with. Actually, you went out "to exercise," but it seemed much more than that. It is very important for you to see your play sessions each day as adventures, not as "exercise," although they are that too.

Adventure suggests new discoveries, doing new things, meeting new people, the unfamiliar. For many overweight people exercise or play has become unfamiliar; in fact, that's the cause of their overweight. So reacquainting yourself with fun activities like cycling, dancing, skipping, the trampoline, perhaps roller skating or ice skating, should give you a series of adventures. I have the same feeling when I occasionally go skiing, because it's an unfamiliar experience for me.

And, of course, when you start on a new activity you are bound to meet people. Often, you'll find that they are starting a new adventure, too, so they will be anxious to share information and their concerns. For one person, to brave the world by jogging through a public street can be a daunting experience; for two people, an exercise in togetherness; for three, a celebration. And you'll find that people starting to exercise, like you, are nice people. They want to help, not criticize. And if they can help you play more, and lose weight while you're doing it, they'll feel good, too. And, of course, you will be helping them. By and large, adventures are better when shared.

You will notice that the activities in the Play Plans include several that move you around your neighborhood. Walking, jogging, cycling and roller skating are examples. These are real adventure exercises, and at least one of them should be regularly included in your Play Plan, because they are your passport to a new world. There are all sorts of things out there that you usually don't see from your car or the bus. As you progress through your plans your range extends, so you can travel farther and see new buildings, new industries, new birds, new animals. Within a few miles of any home or office is a world of unfamiliar scenes waiting to be explored. And if you travel, a further panorama of experiences awaits you. There are the beaches of the world, if you are in Miami or San Diego or Sydney or Cape Town. And so many lakes, small and large to cycle round; and all those cities with rivers to run along: the Thames, the Mississippi, the Danube. Or you may be in a large city. The backstreets of London or New York are always full of life and excitement that is accessible to the visiting walker or runner. Or at other times you may be near mountains or the deserts, near new adventures.

With the entire world accessible to the playful person prepared to move himself around, it does seem rather odd to hear an exercise program described as "boring." It is, after all, the sedentary program, the "go nowhere, see nothing, sit in front of the screen and experience it all secondhand in the privacy of your own living room" plan that is boring. So, if your Play Plan says "cycle five miles," go and see what they are doing with that dredger down by the river, or explore some of those roads behind the school that you've never traveled before.

Play Pals

This may be the most important part of this book. Success with the Play Plans is the vital part of this program, and playing with a friend is the key to success with the Play Plans.

Unquestionably, somewhere there is another human being, male or female, who would be a perfect play pal for you. You both have much to gain and weight to lose. You can support each other, and move together to fitness and lower weight. That person may not be as you imagine him — or her. Don't feel that your pal must be of the same sex — or the same age. All you need is the same goal. An overweight young woman may be the perfect partner for an older, out-of-shape man — or vice versa. But it is important that your physical condition be similar to your partner's. For example, a person capable of cycling 30 miles would not be compatible with a beginner able to cycle only five miles. I wouldn't hesitate to approach an overweight person at work, or on your street, to see if he is interested in forming a partnership for a common goal: reduced weight and increased fitness. You may find a person who can introduce you to tennis, or squash, or running; many overweight people are getting into these sports. You may also be introduced to some quite unexpected area of knowledge while you are exercising. During my lifetime I have run with many different partners, and I am sure we have exchanged a great deal of information. For example, at one time I ran with a Ph.D. student in English, studying *The*

Rape of Lucrece, so, of course, I came to know of the social implications of this Shakespearean poem in some detail. At another period I learned much about California architecture from an architect running partner.

Work As Play

Work as play may be the most difficult concept to swallow. But as our lives become more and more sedentary, the prospect of some burdensome hard work, some polishing or cleaning, may actually acquire attractive features. "Hard work" has never prevented people from deriving great enjoyment — ask the person who has just won the Olympic marathon, or the Nobel Prize. There may be many good activities around the house and garden that normally don't get done, or that you don't do. The mere fact that they are unfamiliar will make them more fun. And remember that many of these tasks are valuable calorie burners, listed in the Play Plans. So don't neglect window cleaning, floor scrubbing or raking leaves as worthwhile play activities. Play music while you clean, and in a few weeks the whole house will look better. If you know you are progressing along your weight-loss plan at the same time, it makes the activity that much more rewarding.

Mix and Match

The Play Plans do not instruct you to do *one* thing: walk, or jog. A variety of equivalent activities is presented. And it is good to try several of them in one month. Walking is probably the easiest and most accessible activity for most overweight people to start with, and at all stages it is important to walk regularly. But try other things, too. Do one activity each day. Fit in some aerobic dancing or skating one day each week, to make a change, an adventure to look forward to. Have one day each week devoted to household chores, and one on the weekend playing in the garden, if you have one. If you can walk all or part of the way to work, that is an excellent way to get regular, useful play. But if not, try walking for 20 to 40 minutes on your lunch hour. Don't do one playful activity only — it is more likely to get boring. But with a menu of activities, and a play pal to keep you company, the "exercise" part of *The California Diet* should be easy and enjoyable.

It All Adds Up

Being overweight is the culmination of a lot of little inactivities. Being slim is the sum of many little activities. Part of the adventure of the Play Plans is seeing how this really operates, and how every little effort to push up the calorie expenditure rate goes to your credit. In the next chapter we will go over some simple ways to burn calories faster, that don't show up on the Play Plans, but they all count. An hour of standing is better than an hour of sitting, an hour of walking is better than an hour of standing, and an hour of jogging is better than an hour of walking. The body keeps count very carefully, and it all goes down in the account book. So think each day how you can "bank" more calories used. Plan your day with that in mind: walk, don't ride; stand, don't sit.

Toward a Playful Future

Seeing weight come steadily down during the year will be a special adventure for most overweight people — an unfamiliar experience. A real feel for the powerful influence of play level on body weight is one of the rewards of finishing the program year. Slim people seem to sense when their activity levels are inadequate, and automatically compensate. The object of the Play Plans is to guide you gradually to healthy levels of play and to leave you as you once were: eager to get out to play each day. Other things came along, and play got squeezed out — perhaps for 30 years. We know what went wrong; we know how to put things right.

6. How To Become a Playful Person

PLAY GRADUALLY

As you start on the play part of *The California Diet*, remember the two keys to success:

• Your activities must be enjoyable. They may become hard work later, but nobody minds hard work when it's fun and play.

• Start playing very slowly, but always progress gradually toward a little more activity each month. Too much exercise, too soon, has caused many people to quit when they could have gone on to become fit and slim. Follow the Play Plans carefully, especially for the first few months! Don't overdo!

Checkup?

Should you check with your physician or other medical adviser before starting on the Play Plans?

The plans are graduated, start at a very low level of intensity and progress slowly. A healthy but overweight individual who is not *extremely* overweight (more than 80 pounds above the maximum of your "ideal" weight range, as stated in Chapter 2) should be able to start on these plans without specific "medical approval." The play activities of the first months are basic activities required to go about our normal lives. Nonetheless, it is a good idea to inform your medical adviser of your intention of slowly losing weight on *The California Diet*, and to invite his opinion of the specific activities you choose. For instance, you *can* do the entire play program by means of walking, which is within the capacity of almost everyone, although this is less fun than mixing activities.

If you are extremely overweight, or know that you suffer from a major disease (heart problem, lung problem, severe arthritis, diabetes, orthopedic problems, or any other major problem), or if you are a heavy smoker, then you should consult your medical adviser before starting this or any other exercise program. He may want to test your health. There are very few conditions where the verdict is "You must do *no* exercise whatever." It is sometimes a question of choosing the *proper* activity (for example, swimming may be best for people with joint problems), and your doctor can assist you here.

When you are on the plans, listen to your body. Most of what you hear will be cheerful news. If your muscles always ache, you are proceeding too fast. If you really hurt, back off and consult your doctor. *If you ever experience severe chest pains while exercising (or at any other time), stop the activity immediately and summon medical aid.*

Types of Play

All types of play and exercise require energy, and so help to control our body weight. But different types of play have different effects on our bodies. The great majority of these effects are beneficial, which is why we should become as playful as possible — it's good for us! Some of the good effects have to do with our long-term health and avoidance of disease: These will be considered in detail in Chapter 8. Other benefits relate to our ability to work and play, and we will look at these now. The most important changes relate to the development of:

• **Endurance** — our ability to keep performing the same activity for prolonged periods. Endurance can be low (poor stamina) or high (good stamina).

• **Strength** — our ability to move or lift weight against gravity. This can be the weight of our own body (running up stairs) or some other weight (repeatedly lifting a barbell). Strength can be little (weak) or great (strong).

• **Flexibility** — how easily we can move the muscles and joints across their maximum normal range of motion without damage or pain. Flexibility can be poor (inflexible) or good (very flexible).

Different types of play develop these attributes to different extents, so while we are becoming more playful, because this is the way to lose and, especially, to control body weight, we might as well improve in these other respects as well. Ideally, a mixture of different sorts of play would best develop endurance, strength and flexibility. And having these three attributes is an important part of "feeling good." People who have little stamina and are weak and inflexible generally don't "feel good." Do you feel good? People who have endurance, strength and flexibility are "fit."

The following table rates many of the major play activities with respect to endurance, strength and flexibility, and some other attributes. At the bottom, for each play type, is a total, giving an idea of the relative value of the different activities. These ratings are quite subjective, and are useful only to classify roughly the different types of play. As I mention constantly, gradualness and enjoyment are the most important factors in selecting your play.

Let's look at a few representative types of play:

Bowling. Lots of fun, but not much else. Bowling involves little moving about and expenditure of energy, so it scores low on all major attributes: endurance, strength and flexibility. However, it is better than watching television!

Weightlifting. Not shown on the table, weightlifting is a "one-thing" sport. It is great for increasing muscular strength and delineation, but it does very little for endurance, especially the important cardiorespiratory endurance. It also does little for weight control. But it is a good form of play, when you're fit enough for it, to *add* to other endurance-promoting sports.

Walking. Walking is a good moderate-level all-around activity. It is much better than weightlifting, but not quite up to the standards of the "big three," bicycling, swimming and running/jogging. But walking is perfect for *starting* your play program, and should be part of everybody's daily play. It's so practical!

Tennis. An "intermediate" exercise, tennis produces moderate endurance and muscle strength, and is superior to running or cycling for flexibility. And a lot of fun!

Swimming, Bicycling, Running/Jogging. You can see from the table why these are the big three! All are good for endurance and strength; swimming is ahead on flexibility and behind on balance. We try to bring one or more of these play activities into your Play Plan as early as possible, consistent with the vital *gradual* approach. Most people with 20 to 80 pounds to lose can start slowly at cycling and swimming, increasing time and playing harder as the months go by. Although running/jogging is (narrowly) at the top of the list of sports, it is not for everyone. If you take to it well, it's an excellent basic sport for weight control. But you should try running only after you've been on your Play Plans for some time (jogging, which is simply slow running, does not appear as a choice until Play Plan F, at the seventh month).

So, in the process of playing away calories, as shown in the Play Plans, we should also acquire as much fitness as we can by mixing our play. And the variety keeps it fun!

RATING FOURTEEN POPULAR SPORTS

Physical Fitness	Running/ Jogging	Bicycling	Swimming
Cardiorespiratory endurance (stamina)	21	19	21
Muscular endurance	20	18	20
Muscular strength	17	16	14
Flexibility	9	9	15
Balance	17	18	12
General Well-Being			
Weight control	21	20	15
Muscle definition	14	15	14
Digestion	13	12	13
Sleep	16	15	16
Total	148	142	140

Physical Fitness	Basketball	Tennis	Calisthenics (Aerobic Dancing)
Cardiorespiratory endurance (stamina)	19	16	10
Muscular endurance	17	16	13
Muscular strength	15	14	16
Flexibility	13	14	19
Balance	16	16	15
General Well-Being			
Weight control	19	16	12
Muscle definition	13	13	18
Digestion	10	12	11
Sleep	12	11	12
Total	134	128	126

Adapted from: Conrad, C. Carson, "How Different Sports Rate in Promoting Physical Fitness."
President's Council on Physical Fitness and Sports, Washington, D.C., U.S. Department of Health,

Skating (Ice or Roller)	Handball/ Squash	Skiing-Nordic (Cross-Country)	Skiing-Alpine (Down-hill)
18	19	19	16
17	18	19	18
15	15	15	15
13	16	14	14
20	17	16	21
17	19	17	15
14	11	12	14
11	13	12	9
15	12	15	12
140	140	139	134

Walking	Golf (with cart or caddy)	Softball	Bowling
13	8	6	5
14	8	8	5
11	9	7	5
7	8	9	7
8	8	7	6
13	6	7	5
11	6	5	5
11	7	8	7
14	6	7	6
102	66	64	51

Education and Welfare, Public Health Service, February 1979. These ratings were computed by averaging the ratings given each sport and exercise by seven physical fitness experts.

The number of calories you burn during your play depends on the sort of play you select, how hard you play, and how heavy you are. It is comforting to know that the heavier you are, the more calories you burn doing the same activity, so some play at the start of your program is particularly helpful to weight loss. Here is a list of activities showing approximately how long it takes to use 100 calories. These figures are for a person weighing 180 pounds playing moderately. If you weigh less, you will burn calories more slowly; if you weigh more, you burn calories more quickly. If you play in a leisurely way, you will burn calories more slowly than indicated; if you play hard, you will burn calories faster. Remember, conditions (temperature, terrain) can influence calorie costs considerably, so use these figures only as a guide.

PLAY ACTIVITY	MINUTES TO BURN 100 CALORIES
Run / Jog (on flat)	9 (5-15)
Climb stairs	10
Saw wood	10
Play racquetball	10
Swim	10 (7-20)
Jump on trampoline	12
Mow lawn	12
Play soccer	13
Roller skate	15
Dance (aerobic)	15
Dig in garden	17
Cycle (on flat)	18 (10-25)
Walk	20
Dance (disco)	20
Play table tennis	20
Play volleyball	20
Clean windows	20
Scrub floors	20
Rake leaves	20

TYPICAL PLAY PLANS

Each Play Plan (pp. 272-277) gives you a selection of activities from which to choose each day. Of course, we could give a single activity (e.g. swimming). This might seem simpler, but then perhaps you don't like swimming, don't have a pool available, can't swim, and so on. As discussed earlier, a variety of play is also desirable to promote all-round fitness and to counteract boredom.

Choose activities from your current month's plan that fit your lifestyle, that you enjoy, and that help to get the work done all at the same time. A player starting with Month 1, Play Plan A, who is just beginning his Calorie Plan for Month 1, might make the choices shown on the next table.

The first two weeks are the choices of Audrey, a woman who works five days a week and lives in a shared home with a friend. Her choices are influenced by her job, her home, and an acquaintance's advice that aerobic dancing is fun. So she gets her *extra* 25 calories per day from walking during the lunch hour, working on the house or garden, and attending the aerobic dance class on Thursday evenings at the local YWCA (the instructor knows that she can't dance the full 30 minutes yet). On Sundays she walks, or swims at the local pool.

The third, fourth, and fifth weeks of Play Plan A were put together by Mary, a woman at home all week with her 1-year-old son. She needs to get to the stores regularly, yet must look after her son, so she takes him with her on a bicycle with a child's seat, strapped in, or carries him to the stores in a shoulder pack. Either way, she exercises while getting the shopping done. Mary also has to do the housework, and so chooses some extra window cleaning and scrubbing, with music from the radio. Not only is she filling her 25-calorie quota this way, her home starts to look better than it used to. Curiously, she meets Audrey at the aerobic dance class on Thursday night, when her husband looks after their son; they all meet again at the local swimming pool on Sunday. Both women are carefully following the plan in the very gradual way that will keep them on course for the entire year. They agree to meet regularly on Thursdays at the aerobic dance class, and compare notes about their weight loss.

━━━━━━━━━━AUDREY━━━━━━━━━━

	DAY	WEEK 1		WEEK 2
MONDAY	1	Walk from office to post office on lunch hour (3 blocks)	8	Walk to stores in lunch hour (3 blocks)
TUESDAY	2	Clean windows before work (wake up earlier: 6 minutes)	9	Clean windows before work (6 minutes)
WEDNESDAY	3	Walk with friend on lunch hour (3 blocks)	10	Walk with friend on lunch hour (3 blocks)
THURSDAY	4	Aerobic dance class at YWCA (5 minutes) in evening	11	Aerobic dance class at YWCA (5 minutes) in evening
FRIDAY	5	Walk to stores on lunch hour (3 blocks)	12	Walk to stores on lunch hour (3 blocks)
SATURDAY	6	Rake leaves or scrub floor (6 minutes)	13	Scrub floor or clean windows (6 minutes)
SUNDAY	7	Walk in neighborhood, early morning (3 blocks)	14	Swim in local pool (3 minutes)

MARY

	WEEK 3		WEEK 4		WEEK 5
15	Cycle to stores with child in carrier (1 mile)	22	Cycle to stores with child in carrier (1 mile)	29	Cycle to stores with child in carrier (1 mile)
16	Clean windows to music (6 minutes)	23	Clean windows to music (6 minutes)	30	Clean windows to music (6 minutes)
17	Walk to store with child in shoulder pack (3 blocks)	24	Walk to store with child in shoulder pack (3 blocks)		
18	Aerobic dance class at YWCA (5 minutes) in evening	25	Aerobic dance class at YWCA (5 minutes) in evening		
19	Scrub floor to music (6 minutes)	26	Scrub floor to music (6 minutes)		
20	Cycle to store with child in carrier (1 mile)	27	Cycle to store with child in carrier (1 mile)		
21	Swim in local pool with family (3 minutes)	28	Walk in neighborhood, with family (3 blocks)		

TYPICAL PLAY PLAN "A"

25

	DAY	WEEK 1		WEEK 2
MONDAY	1	Walk 1½ miles on lunch hour. Cycle to see friend in evening (26 minutes)	8	Walk 1½ miles on lunch hour. Cycle to see friend in evening (26 minutes)
TUESDAY	2	Walk 1½ miles on lunch hour. Cycle to and from work (26 minutes)	9	Walk 1½ mile on lunch hour. Cycle to and from work (26 minutes)
WEDNESDAY	3	Walk 1½ miles on lunch hour. Walk to wrk (1½ miles); ride back with friend	10	Walk 1½ miles on lunch hour. Cycle to see friend in evening (26 minutes)
THURSDAY	4	Walk 1½ miles on lunch hour. Aerobic dance class at YWCA (24 minutes in evening)	11	Walk 1½ miles on lunch hour. Aerobic dance class at YWCA (24 minutes) in evening
FRIDAY	5	Walk 1½ miles on lunch hour. Walk to work (1½ miles); ride back with friend	12	Walk 1½ miles on lunch hour. Walk to work (1½ miles), ride back with friend
SATURDAY	6	Walk 1½ miles before breakfast. Dance (disco) for 24 minutes	13	Walk 1½ miles before breakfast. Dance (disco) for 24 minutes
SUNDAY	7	Walk 1½ miles before dinner. Dig in the garden for 26 minutes	14	Walk 1½ miles before dinner. Saw wood for 15 minutes

WEEK 3		WEEK 4		WEEK 5
15	Walk 1½ miles before breakfast. Trampoline to music (18 minutes) afternoon	22	Walk 1½ miles before dinner. Trampoline to music (18 minutes) after-noon	29	Walk 1½ miles before breakfast. Trampoline to music (18 minutes) afternoon
16	Walk 1½ miles before dinner. Trampoline to music (18 minutes) afternoon	23	Walk 1½ miles before breakfast. Trampoline to music (18 minutes) afternoon	30	Walk 1½ miles before dinner Trampoline to music (18 minutes) afternoon
17	Walk 1½ miles before breakfast. Trampoline to music (18 minutes) afternoon	24	Walk 1½ miles before breakfast. Trampoline to music (18 minutes) afternoon		
18	Walk 1½ miles before breakfast. Aerobic dance class at YWCA (24 minutes) in evening	25	Walk 1½ miles before dinner. Aerobic dance class at YWCA (24 minutes) in evening		**TYPICAL PLAY PLAN "H"**
19	Walk 1½ miles before dinner. Trampoline to music (18 minutes) afternoon	26	Walk 1½ miles before breakfast. Trampoline to music (18 minutes) afternoon		300
20	Walk 1½ miles before dinner. Swim 15 minutes in afternoon	27	Walk 1½ miles before breakfast. Swim 15 minutes in afternoon		
21	Walk 1½ miles before breakfast. Roller skate for 24 minutes	28	Walk 1½ miles before dinner. Roller skate for 24 minutes		

The next table shows our two ladies one year later. Now they are on Play Plan H, and using 300 extra calories each day. They have carefully linked their Calorie Plans to their Play Plans, and both are eating more now than they were one year ago. Audrey has lost 35 pounds, and Mary 28 pounds. Both are delighted, and both are now very fit.

At this stage, both Audrey and Mary are walking 1½ miles every day. Audrey does this on her lunch hour, combined with visiting the stores; it has become a pleasant routine. Sometimes office friends join her. On the weekends Audrey walks before breakfast or before dinner. Mary gets her mile-and-a-half walk in either before breakfast or when her husband returns from work, about 5:30 p.m. She uses the evening walks to do some grocery shopping, which she carries home. "I just can't believe that a year ago I would sit indoors for days on end and never go out for a walk," Mary confides to Audrey.

Audrey adds to her walking by cycling quite often; she has a new 10-speed bike. It gets her to work some days, and takes her to see friends. A new feature of Audrey's life is dancing on Saturday nights. It's a nice social occasion — and it uses calories too! With all this extra play, Audrey's garden gets neglected, so she attends to that on Sunday mornings. On Thursday evenings it is time for aerobic dancing. Audrey and Mary dance side-by-side and know all the routines. They go through the 30-minute session (well, 24 minutes dancing, counting breaks). "That's another 150 calories," Mary says. "Do you remember when we did just five minutes?"

Mary has found some play activities that she really enjoys to get her daily 300 calories. Being at home all week, she had to come up with something that was fun and possible to do at home. Her husband bought her a small trampoline and now she bounces on that most weekdays to her favorite radio program, or to records. Mary still swims for 15 minutes on Saturdays. Her latest play: she roller-skates! Each Sunday morning she joins some young neighbors. Says it makes her feel like a kid again! Her plan doesn't allow for any extra housework; but Mary feels so lively these days that the polishing and cleaning get done much faster. All part of being fit, she says.

Audrey and Mary agree that the one-year plan went by fast. It was so gradual and so easy, it's hard to believe that one year ago they were each 30 pounds or so heavier, totally out of shape and eating *less!* "Just getting out of the house regularly was the key," says Mary. "And out of the office," echoes Audrey.

Play Records

Keep a record of your play right from the first day. A good idea is to use a blank calendar of the type that has room to record a few sentences each day of each month. Write down the type and amount of play you do each day, and any other brief notes of interest to you — who you play with or the weather conditions. But keep it brief so that it takes only a moment to update your record each day: Don't let it become a burden. Keep your play record near your bathroom scale or on your bedside table, so you can't miss it. The record helps you to check how closely you are keeping to the Play Plan, and whether you are doing too little or too much. It is also very revealing later in your program to look back and see how much more you can now accomplish, and how fit you have become.

How Hard Should I Play?

How hard should I play? The best answer is "Whatever level of activity makes you feel good about your play session, and eager to come back tomorrow for the next session." Remember that any additional energy expenditure, at any level, will burn calories and is going to help you control weight. Walking very slowly for an hour is about equivalent to walking very fast for a half-hour, from the point of view of calories used.

But there's another aspect to play that determines how fit you become. You can estimate whether your play is helping you to improve endurance and strength by measuring your exercise heart rate. To do this, you stop your play (for example, you would have to stop cycling or stop at the end of the swimming pool) and immediately measure your rate by counting beats for 10 seconds at your neck (place your first two fingers firmly on one side of your throat until you detect your pulse, then count the number of beats in 10 seconds, using a watch displaying seconds). This takes a little practice, and the rate you get in 10 seconds falls rapidly as soon as you stop exercising, so you must start counting immediately upon stopping the activity. Multiply your count by six to get your exercise heart rate in beats per minute.

Now you need to know whether your heart rate while playing is too low, too high or "about right." If it is too high, you may be overdoing it, and should probably play a little more gently. If it is too low, you will not be getting fitter, although you will be helping your weight control; consider playing a little more energetically, so long as you continue to feel good. To be "about right," your exercise heart rate should be in the target range, which you can calculate like this:

- Write down 220
- Write down your age (say, 40)

- Subtract your age from 220:
  e.g. $220 - 40 = 180$
- Multiply the number you obtain by 0.65 and also by 0.85:
  e.g. $180 \times 0.65 = 117$
  $180 \times 0.85 = 153$

- Your *target range* is 117 to 153 beats per minute.

This gives you a rough indication of whether or not your play level is making you fitter. Since this method is approximate, you could round off the figures in the example above to 120 to 155. So, if you are 40 and when cycling you find your exercise heart rate is 170, you should slow down a bit. If your rate immediately after stopping cycling is 105, for instance, you can afford to pedal faster!

I must emphasize again that this system is simply an attempt to answer the very common question "Am I putting enough effort into my play, or too much?" But remember that how you feel is the best indicator for you, so "listen to your body."

Tips on Increasing Calorie Use

The Play Plans are an attempt to indicate about how much extra play you need to get the better of your weight problem. It is not simply a matter of losing the excess fat you have accumulated over the years; the important thing is that you learn gradually to become more playful, and unconsciously play for some time each day. You should feel something is missing if you don't. When you get to the levels of plans H, I and J, you will start to regulate your weight automatically, with the need for much less conscious thought about how much you eat. You will, in fact, now be eating quite a bit more than you once did, when you weighed *more*.

In addition to the activities described for each day of the Play Plans, there are many other things you can do to increase your calorie use during the day. When we talk about "counting calories," what should we be thinking about? How many calories are in every little thing we eat during the day? Well, true, but equally important, and probably more important, is thinking about every little thing we do during the day. Count the calories in your everyday life, and spend, spend, spend! What has made you overweight is the saving, hoarding, miserly attitude of your body over the years. Every spare calorie has been hoarded away as fat. Now is the time to splurge. Be profligate with your calories every chance you get:

- Stand while talking on the telephone, instead of sitting.
- Stand on the bus or train, instead of sitting.
- Use the rest room farthest from your work area. If it is up several flights of stairs, great! Revel in those extra calories used;

mentally check them off as another little victory in the war.

• Park your car as far away in the parking lot as you can and walk in. (Even if the car stands lonely in the far corner of the lot).

• Avoid elevators and escalators whenever you can. A red light should flash whenever you see one. Develop a reputation for always taking the stairs; others will join you.

• Don't ask someone to bring something to you (a file, coffee). Go and get it yourself, and mentally mark down those few extra calories spent.

• When the telephone rings, promptly walk to the most distant extension you can use. Ten yards are better than two when you answer the telephone 5000 times a year!

• Your child can help you lose weight! Carry him in a shoulder pack instead of pushing a stroller or using the car for short journeys.

Watching television is the single leisure time activity that the largest number of people do every day (75 percent). The amount of fat that settles down on the frame of Americans each year while they are innocently seated watching the soap operas is staggering, to be measured in thousands of tons. Here are some things to do while you are watching (well, peeking at) television:

• Ride a stationary bike
• Polish shoes
• Stretch
• Polish silver
• Wash dishes
• Lift weights
• Jump rope
• Bounce on a trampoline.

All of these activities will increase the calorie cost of your television watching.

The success of your one-year weight-loss program can be increased greatly by doing these various things, some using large numbers of calories, others tiny numbers, as well as the main play activities. It is a question of seizing every opportunity to burn a few extra calories, and it all adds up quickly. This is exactly what most slim people do during their days. Delight in finding new ways to burn a few more calories, ways that have eluded you before. (Hint: try standing up for the rest of this chapter).

Clothing and Equipment

There seems to be very little relationship between the cost and complexity of play equipment and clothing, and a person's play habits. But you will need some clothing and equipment to do justice to your play, and to enjoy it. Here are some hints in often-encountered areas.

Warm-up suit. The warm-up suit is probably the best single investment you can make, whatever sort of play you enjoy. It's useful for all sports. Be sure it is easy to wash and dry, and that the bottoms don't tend to come down when you move around. The new suits are bright and attractive and make you feel good about playing. After your first few months on the plans, think about getting a second warm-up suit. Soon you will need a smaller one. (Note: Never wear rubber suits or other garments).

Shoes. A vast array of sports shoes in every conceivable style and color now awaits your choice. Most important: good fit! Try them on in the store with the socks you will normally wear (thin cotton socks are usually most comfortable). Be sure both shoes are big enough. A common fault is buying shoes that seem to fit in the store, but pinch or rub when you wear them to play. If in doubt, take the larger size, but be sure your feet don't slip around in the shoes, either. Remember that your feet will swell somewhat when blood circulation increases during exercise. Comfortable shoes are vital for enjoyment of so many types of play. "Running shoes" are good for walking, using the trampoline, volleyball, and playing around the house. Get expert advice from a specialty store when buying footwear for special types of play: hiking boots, roller skates, ice skates, ski boots, soccer shoes. Attend to your feet and don't give yourself this excuse to quit: "My feet hurt."

Socks. Cotton socks are good to absorb sweat and thus reduce risk of blisters while walking, running, cycling, and so on. Use the special socks made for hiking, skating and skiing.

Tops, Shorts and Bras. Cotton T-shirts are useful for a variety of types of play. Be comfortable, and don't overdress when it is warm: We are designed to sweat. Synthetic shorts (nylon mainly) with built-in pants (his and hers) are very convenient. Get a good fit to avoid chafing. A bra providing firm support is essential for women. It is well worth the investment of a few dollars to try several makes, and seek advice when looking for a suitable exercise bra. Avoid seams and metal parts, and look out for chafing.

Gloves and a Wool Cap. Gloves and a hat are vital for cold weather play outdoors.

Bicycle. If you don't own a bicycle or have only an old one-speed or three-speed, and if you like cycling, consider making the investment in a good 10-speed. By using different gears you can get up and down the hills faster, and 10-speeds are usually much lighter than standard one- and three-speeds. Find a good bike shop and an attentive sales clerk. Have the bike fitted with standard handlebars (without the U-shaped curve) and a comfortable seat. We want you to stay with it! Later, you may want to change handlebars to the maes (curved down type), change to a smaller, firmer seat and use toe clips and toe straps; but adapt the bike for comfort initially, so that you can start getting the play miles in. Include a bike rack that will accommodate whatever purse, briefcase, or jacket you normally travel with, especially if you will cycle to and from work. Make the bike useful in your life, so that you will ride it often.

Trampoline. There are many good mini-trampolines available for home use, starting at around $100. Mini-trampolines are a good play investment if you *must* stay indoors much of the time to look after children, or if you just can't bring yourself to exercise outdoors yet. They're excellent to use to music — radio or tape-recorded. Get a trampoline with as large a rebounding area as possible, and be sure the metal parts are well padded.

Stationary bicycle. A very good investment is the stationary bicycle, if you are sure you will be spending a lot of play time indoors. Better models cost $250. This is a useful way to get extra play while doing something else — watching television, or reading the paper. This play method has drawbacks compared to walking, or riding outdoors on your 10-speed. Riders of stationary bicycles do not meet people, or see the world!

Skates, Rackets, Skis. If you're new to skating, racket sports or skiing, consult a good sports store or, better still, find a veteran player of the sport for his advice on purchases.

Togetherness

Exercise is a game where any number can play. Take running, for instance. Some players love solitude, and like to run alone with only their thoughts. A few runners have even traversed the United States alone, a feat requiring 80 pounds of fat and a fair amount of self-assurance. But runners can also be gregarious, and most love to play together. San Francisco's annual Bay to Breakers race attracts some 50,000 runners who traverse the city in a carnival atmosphere, many in costume. This is the largest American play event (in terms of numbers of players); but races with several thousand entrants are commonplace now.

For many people starting to play again after many years of unplayfulness, company is very reassuring and just what they need.

Play Pals. If you can find that ideal partner, play will be more fun: a friend, neighbor, or colleague who wants to lose weight too. You have many millions from whom to choose! Perhaps the man in your apartment building who needs to lose weight, or the new woman at work with 30 pounds to shed is right for you. You can support each other, encourage each other to get out and play in foul weather, share information, laugh about it all. What might be a grim, individual battle alone, becomes a fun adventure with a friend. Sound corny? Ask people who have done this and made lifelong friends. Here is a truth you will learn: A colleague who is rather formal, unsympathetic in the hallway or at the staff meeting, will become quite extroverted and easy going when he is climbing hills on a bicycle with you, or lining up for the first aerobic dance class. "Shared adversity," even a little, rather contrived adversity, does wonders for togetherness. We are, after all, in this together; and if we can win the weight-loss battle together, holding hands, well, good for us!

Little Groups. The world is full of sport clubs, and many can help the overweight person beginning to play. How do you find out about bicycles? Join a cycling club. How do you learn aerobic dancing? Join the YMCA, YWCA or your town recreation program; they probably have regular classes. There are always experienced people in your neighborhood who know the answers to these questions, and most of them are eager to offer advice. Ask around at work: There may be a walking group, or swimming group or cycling group already in existence that you don't know about. Groups of runners are always forming where there is interest. Most conventions that last longer than a day will soon produce groups of runners, jogging and stretching in the hotel lobby.

Big Groups. There is information, inspiration and advice to be gained from national organizations. The Sierra Club, for instance, has done a great deal for weight control in America, not to mention our environment. There are all sorts of organizations for cyclists, walkers, soccer players, runners, the list goes on. The Fifty-Plus Runners Association appeals to the older fitness-conscious person. The new group shares an interest in fitness through running as a way toward a "New Deal" for the over-fifty crowd. Magazines on sport abound. They'll provide information, social contacts and help generate enthusiasm.

Warmup, Cooldown

For many types of play, a warmup is not necessary. You needn't go through a stretching routine before walking three blocks or cycling slowly for a few miles. But for some forms of play, especially in the later Play Plans, gentle stretching is a good idea to let your muscles and joints know that play time is coming. Apart from this, a daily stretching routine is good for flexibility and "feeling good." Some points about warmup and stretching:

• Do the stretches regularly. Once each day is best.
• Stretch before vigorous exercises like running/jogging, playing soccer, skating.
• Stretch when you are just sitting around watching television.
• Stretch slowly, without bouncing. Don't force muscles, or they become even more tight.
• Stretching should not be painful. Remember our golden rule: gradualness. Stretch just a little today, more next week, much more next month. When you are overweight, your muscles may be quite out of shape. Give them at least a few weeks to get back in condition. But do a little, every day.
• Avoid exercises that involve deep-knee bends (they cause knee problems), arching the back in the unnatural direction (they worsen or cause back problems) or make you red in the face (they raise blood pressure excessively). Push-ups and pull-ups should be avoided until you are much fitter.
• If you are one of many millions who is overweight, and has arthritis or other back and joint problems, consult your medical adviser about stretching and play in general. Remember that regular exercise is usually very beneficial in those conditions, and improves the mobility and use of joints. Regular back exercises have worked wonders for back-pain sufferers, and should, for many, be part of the daily routine for people with back pain. Remember, too, that as you lose weight your back pain is very likely to improve, because overweight contributes to the condition.

Here is a set of six moderately strenuous exercises. You can do them standing up, so you don't have to get muddy if you are in the park on a wet day and feel like stretching. You can stretch most of your major muscles this way in a five- to 10-minute session.

Some people like to stretch *after* their play session, (cool down), as well as before. You can use the same set of six exercises that you use for warming up.

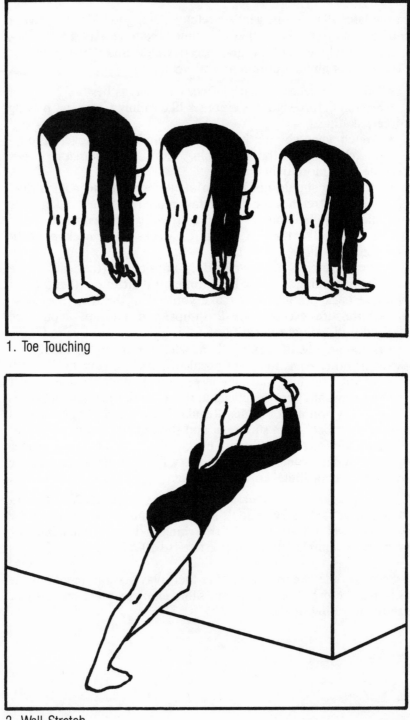

1. Toe Touching

2. Wall Stretch

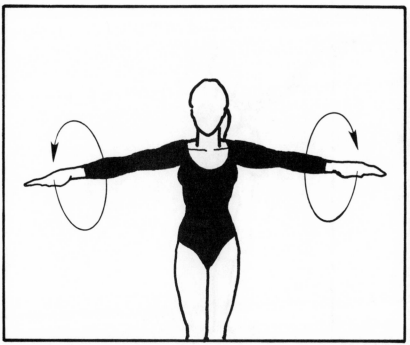

3. Arm Rotations

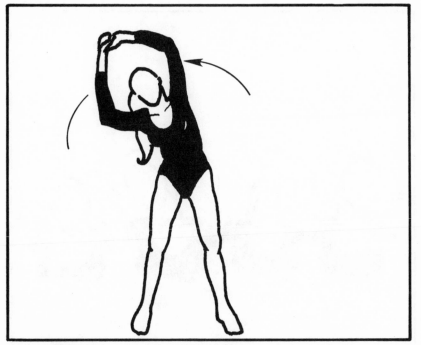

4. Side Bends

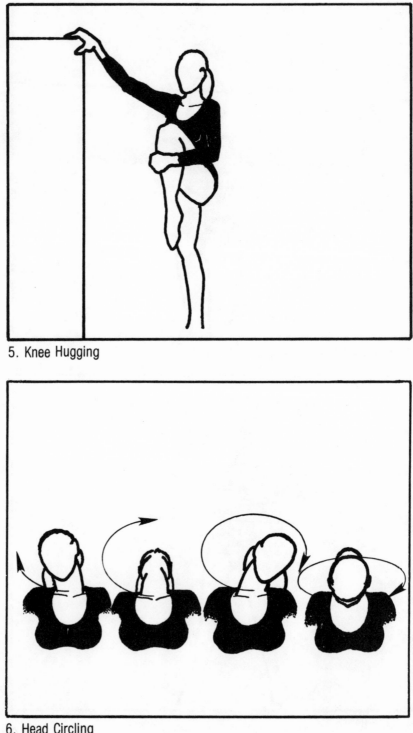

5. Knee Hugging

6. Head Circling

Things to Watch Out For

Like all other worthwhile human endeavors, play has some hazards and it is best to head them off whenever we can. For people on *The California Diet*, the strenuousness of play will not be high for many months, so some of the possible hazards are remote for you until you become very fit, beyond Play Plan H.

Major hazards to be aware of are as follows, in approximate order of importance to the overweight player.

Road accidents. By no means confined to players, this is a hazard to which we should all be alert. Studies of road accidents involving walkers, runners and cyclists, who must share the highways with cars and trucks, show that the important points are: Walk, run or cycle only one abreast on the roadway. Cyclists, use bike paths where available, or ride *with* traffic. Walkers and joggers, face the oncoming traffic. Avoid the roads at night. If you must use the roads when it is dark, wear reflective clothing. Cyclists, watch especially for vehicles turning right at intersections when you are on their near side. Cyclists, wear protective helmets.

Swimming accidents. Do you swim adequately for the distance you are attempting? Observe posted warnings at lakes, rivers and the ocean. Watch out for motor boats.

Personal attack. Avoid walking, jogging or cycling alone in lonely places at night, or near known hazardous areas. Go with your play pal, or else stay in areas where there are usually other people within sight. Carry a "shriek alarm," a device that emits a high-pitched noise when activated.

Heat and humidity. People exercising at high levels for extended periods should consider the hazards of heat and humidity. Excessive loss of sweat without adequate fluid replacement can lead to disorientation and even heat stroke, as body temperature climbs in hot, humid weather. Avoid exercising hard when it is very hot (above 80°F) or humid.

Stop at once if you feel disoriented in hot weather.

Drink plenty of fluids before, during and after your play sessions. This is good practice, whatever the weather.

Heart Problems. Some 500,000 heart attack deaths occur in the United States each year. It is not surprising that some occur during play. If you are in generally good health, with no known heart problems, your risk of having a heart attack during exercise is extremely low, but it is not an impossibility. The same is true for watching television, driving a car or any other activity. The difference is that regular exercise favorably influences risk factors so that your *overall risk* of heart attack at any time is reduced (see Chapter 8).

Injuries. As you start to use your body again, there is a chance of injury to muscles, tendons and ligaments. Many extremely minor "injuries" in active people (and animals) are felt as twinges that come, are rapidly repaired by the body, and are gone next day. This is all part of the natural repair process in a fit individual. When you have been inactive for many years, the chances of an injury that stays with you for days or weeks is increased as you start to play. The best answer to this is to start playing very slowly, which, of course, is another reason why the Play Plans start at a very modest level and build up very slowly, month by month. If you get an injury, ease off for a few days and it will likely go away by itself: You were probably overdoing it.

If an injury persists, read some of the excellent articles listed in the Reference section, and get advice from veterans at the particular game you are playing.

An injury that is severe, or persists for many weeks, deserves attention by a sportsmedicine specialist. Here are some general observations on injuries:

1. Of the types of play mentioned in the Play Plans, walking and swimming are least likely to produce injuries. Cycling, aerobic dancing, tennis and trampoline are intermediate. Downhill skiing is most likely to produce injuries, although these can be minimized with proper equipment and care.

2. Sore muscles are very common when starting any new play. Take a hot bath. You will feel better. Remember gradualness.

3. Use an ice pack on new injuries (first 48 hours) to limit swelling. Use heat on old injuries.

4. Many people who are starting to play after years of inactivity will reactivate old injuries, (e.g., "bad knees" from high school basketball or football). Start very slowly and, if old injuries persist, change your play accordingly. Jogging may *not* be for you. People with long-standing bad backs often find swimming best-suited for them.

5. Knee pain ("runner's knee") is the most common injury to joggers. Check shoes for uneven wear, run on flat, smooth surfaces and avoid running up and down steep hills.

6. Use appropriate protective equipment at all times: a helmet when cycling; knee pads and gloves when skating; goggles when playing racquetball; reflective clothing if exercising on roads at night.

7. Concentrate on the prevention — not cure — of injuries.

8. If the catalog of possible injuries seems long to you, remember that many millions of Americans, having tried regular play for years, willingly accept the risk of occasional injury in exchange for all the benefits of exercise. "But, surely watching television is free of hazards?'' For all the hazards resulting from too much television-watching in the seated position, see Chapter 8.

There are also a number of minor hazards that you may encounter as you set out to become a more playful person. Here are some hints, but each sport has its own list, its own solutions.

Athlete's foot. Athlete's foot is a common fungal infection causing redness and itching irritation between the toes. To prevent it, dry feet thoroughly and use an anti-fungal powder (spray cans are convenient) after every shower, if you are very prone to the infection.

Blisters. Blisters are very common on the feet when you are not used to physical activity (walking, jogging, skating,) and especially in hot weather. Keep your feet dry (cotton socks), because wet skin blisters easily. Shoes that fit well (not too tight!) are essential to minimize blisters. A large blister often feels less painful if the fluid is removed by puncturing with a flame-sterilized needle. Keep the feet clean while blisters are healing.

Chafing. Chafing can be a problem for new players. Watch for tight clothing (underarms, crotch). Use adhesive plaster where necessary, and apply Vaseline where friction occurs.

Dogs. I think we should be nice to dogs. For many people, their dog is their best play pal, always ready to go out to play. A jogger who sallies forth armed to the teeth with chains and Mace, in the event he should meet an elderly dachshund, seems rather absurd to me. Dogs have more to fear from us than we from them.

Admittedly, walkers, runners and cyclists are occasionally bitten by dogs (I have not been bitten by a dog even after 40 years of running on four continents, perhaps because I always talk nicely to dogs). If you *are* bitten, try to determine whether the dog has been protected recently against rabies. In some foreign countries, where canine rabies is more common, greater precautions are warranted.

Frostbite. Frostbite creeps up on you in cold weather. Keep the more vulnerable hands, ears, face and feet covered when you are walking, jogging or cycling and the wind-chill factor is high.

Insects. Unplayful people tend to forget that we share the world with many interesting insects. As you advance through the Play Plans you will meet more insects. If you swallow one as you play, add two calories.

Poisonous plants. Poison oak and poison ivy can be a problem for players who tromp through the woods. Be aware of the telltale identifying characteristics of these plants, and avoid them like the plague as you walk or run. If you think you have been contaminated, take a shower immediately after you return from your play, and use plenty of soap.

Sun Exposure. Wear thin, light-colored clothing to protect you from too much sun; a hat helps protect the head and eyes. Use sun screen. Get your tan gradually. Risk of skin cancer increases with increased exposure to the sun. But most people like the sun on their bodies, so this is another personal decision we have to make: a nice tan now, or increased risk of skin cancer later. Be moderate!

Warts. If you start to use changing rooms and showers more often as you play more, your risk of acquiring warts (little hard lumps on the skin on the bottom of the feet) will increase. These usually grow extremely slowly, but if they occur they are best removed by a professional early before they become well-established. They can also infect your family via the bathroom floor. Inspect your feet occasionally for warts.

Weather. Playing in weather throughout the four seasons is one of the delights of outdoor activity. But avoid starting your Play Plans in extremes of weather. To start Plan A outdoors in Minneapolis in January, or in Phoenix, Arizona, in July, would be stretching any new player's dedication to the limit. Give yourself a chance and start in fair weather.

7. Link Your Eating
to Your Play

Most of the immensely popular diets of the past 10 years, during which time sedentary America has continued to gain weight, have been aimed at reduction of food intake, and the anxious counting of calories *eaten*. *The California Diet* is concerned with diet, because its quality has a lot to do with health. Also, a temporary restriction of calories is necessary to remove accumulated fat from the overweight body in a reasonably short period of time. But as you can see, this program gives great emphasis to calorie expenditure, and the joyful counting of calories *used*.

In *The California Diet*, reduced calorie intakes are part of the *treatment* for the condition that the overweight person has acquired. These low-calorie diets are *not* the preventive measure — it is the Play Plans! Most popular diets provide only a treatment — dieting. It is as if we constantly contracted measles and treated the problem by applying lotion to the spots. An attack on the underlying cause — by widespread vaccination and isolation of sufferers in the case of measles — should accompany the treatment. Similarly, many people will be intermittently dieting forever if they don't tackle the underlying cause — inadequate play.

Why Does Increased Play Work?

We have seen that play satisfies some primeval need, providing a combination of excitement and fun. High levels of play constitute "exercise," and exercise is associated with a long list of health benefits, as described in Chapter 8. Play can also improve our cardiorespiratory endurance (heart and lung) and muscular strength, making us fit, and better able to perform and enjoy many of life's activities.

In addition, the active, playful person reaches and maintains a desirable, reasonably low body fat content: We would say he is usually "slim." Precisely why the weight is maintained still eludes us to some extent. It probably has to do with the loss of the heat-insulating fat layer, resulting in more rapid loss of heat calories; an increased muscle mass, providing more calorie-burning tissue, and an increased resting metabolic rate per pound of muscle, allowing the playful person to burn calories faster even when resting. The very active person increases his caloric intake to compensate for these changes, and for the caloric cost of the play itself. Now he could easily overdo it and eat *too much more,* so that he remains fat, or even gets fatter. *The point is that he doesn't.*

There is a mechanism (area) in the brain of man and in higher animals, popularly know as the appestat, that helps to regulate the amount we eat in relation to our need for food. There are probably other mechanisms that contribute to this balancing process. It is certainly not a simple mechanism. The appestat seems to function much more precisely at "high calorie through-puts"; that is, when a high play level is balanced by high food intake level, as must inevitably happen. On the other hand, the mechanism seems much less precise, with a tendency to err on the side of encouraging a *fraction* too much food intake, when the calorie through-put is low; that is, when a low play level is accompanied by a relatively low food intake. As we have seen, even that very small positive calorie balance accumulates over the years to produce the excess fat you don't want. We were almost certainly intended by nature to be much more active than we have recently become, and hence to eat more than we currently do. Perhaps, then, it is not surprising that the appestat mechanism doesn't work very well for some of us. We may have a control mechanism designed for the old, high-powered model body built into the new low-powered model, and it isn't really suitable.

The public is still told, even by experts, information similar to what follows: "Exercise has the added benefit of decreasing appetite, so it actually makes dieting easier." This is not true, or the exerciser would gradually fade away to nothing. In fact, typical modern weight-losers who have adopted high play levels, such as runners and tennis players, eat considerably more calories than fatter, less playful people (see Reference section). A better way to describe the situation, I believe, is as follows: "Exercise has the added benefit of *increasing* appetite, while simultaneously improving the precision of the appetite-regulating mechanism, leading to an exquisite balance between energy intake and energy output, and usually a desirable body fat content."

Let us not be unduly distressed if we don't know the precise mechanism of good things that happen to us. When Edward Jenner discovered in England, in 1796, that vaccination with cowpox would prevent the scourge of smallpox, it was no great matter to those who avoided the disease that the mechanism of the vaccination process remained obscure for many years. So it is with weight control: For whatever reasons, increasing activity level works for most people!

Link Your Eating to Your Play!

Linking your eating to your play, then, is really what weight control is all about, for most people. The beautifully balanced linking process takes place automatically when your play level is high enough, keeping your weight where you want it.

If you have a bad month on your Play Plans — perhaps you get sick, or the weather is terrible, or you become extremely busy — then you will not lose the weight predicted. If you don't follow the Play Plans, the program will not work (it isn't magic, like some diets!). What to do? You could compensate for playing less by eating less than your Calorie Plan allows. But this is in effect slipping back toward the old one-sided "dieting-only" approach that seldom works for long. The best attitude to a "bad play month" is to accept the lower weight loss you experience that month, and get back on track with your Play Plans as soon as you can. Or you could repeat a month, giving you a 13-month "year" for the total program. My point is that the habit of relying on more extreme dieting *without* play is a bad one, and you should not encourage it!

So, link your eating to your play, and remember: When in doubt, concentrate on the play!

8. The Health Benefits of Play

Increased play is encouraged in *The California Diet* because it is the key to successful long-term weight control — the slim person's secret. Happily, an active life brings with it a host of other health benefits that sometimes have nothing to do with slimness. Scientific knowledge of the benefits of regular exercise has grown apace, in recent years, with America's "exercise explosion." There was no point in spending money on exercise research in 1960, because, I was often told, "Americans will never do any." We have a great deal more to learn about the health consequences of regular exercise, partly because research in this field is difficult, lengthy and costly. Also, exercise has been something of a "Cinderella subject," overshadowed by investigative work on her sisters — ugly or otherwise — diet and drugs.

Chapter 8 takes you on a very brief, guided tour of health areas where regular play activities appear to have a positive influence. It is only reasonable for you to inspect the bill of goods before embarking on the Play Plans. I think you will agree that you get much more for money (or should I say calories?) spent than simply easier weight control.

You will notice that we leap around among several different topics — not neglecting the health of the mind. This is because regular play is now known to benefit many areas of our health. In this respect exercise is unique among health practices; it is the "all-purpose health improver." If you feel inclined to read more in any specific area, you will find selected source material in the Reference section.

FITNESS

Perhaps the most predictable effect of an exercise or "play" program in scientific studies has been an increase in fitness in those who play. The effect is detectable at rather modest levels of play. We see the end result as improved endurance and strength. What actually happens? Big increases occur in the muscle content of the enzymes that enable the muscles to operate. The blood supply to the muscles, through the minute capillaries, also increases. Look at the leg of a world-class marathon runner and it does not appear to be any different from the leg of a sedentary person. It is slimmer and a little more muscular, but inside it is totally different — an extremely efficient, almost tireless energy-producing "factory" compared to the sedentary, easily tired leg. When we think of the performance of the marathon runner, I suppose we should not be surprised that he or she has developed superior equipment. It is not that they were superior to begin with, either. They got that way through proper exercise.

At the other end of the play apparatus is the heart, functioning to supply the exercising muscles with blood, containing fuel and oxygen. To produce a fit individual, all systems must be "go." A good heart and feeble body muscles will get us nowhere, and vice versa. The fit heart is also very different from the unfit heart, and again, training brings about the change. The heart of the regular exerciser tends to be larger than the heart of the sedentary person, but the important difference lies in the amount of blood that the heart can pump through the body with each beat, which is known as the "stroke volume." The chamber of the heart responsible for pumping blood to the general circulation is the muscular *left ventricle*. The amount of blood pumped with a single beat depends on the volume of the left ventricle, and especially on the degree to which it empties when maximally contracted. The left ventricle of a well trained, fit person can contract most effectively, expelling more of the total blood in the chamber than is possible for the less efficient heart of the sedentary person. The result (as shown in the diagram) is a larger amount of blood pumped with each beat (larger stroke volume) for the fit person.

We can look at the consequences of a large stroke volume for a person at rest and when playing hard. When resting, the stroke volume remains high, so the fit person needs fewer beats each minute than the unfit person to provide the amount of blood used by the resting body. So there is a drop in the *resting heart rate* as a person becomes fitter. This is another highly predictable consequence of a training program undertaken by an unfit person. There is one school of thought that holds that the heart is capable of only so many beats, and therefore a slow heart rate during much of the day is an advantage, since the apparatus is likely to have a longer useful life! There is little evidence for this, but if there is any truth in it the active person must have an advantage.

When the fit person is playing hard, the larger stroke volume still operates, so that a much larger volume of blood can be provided to

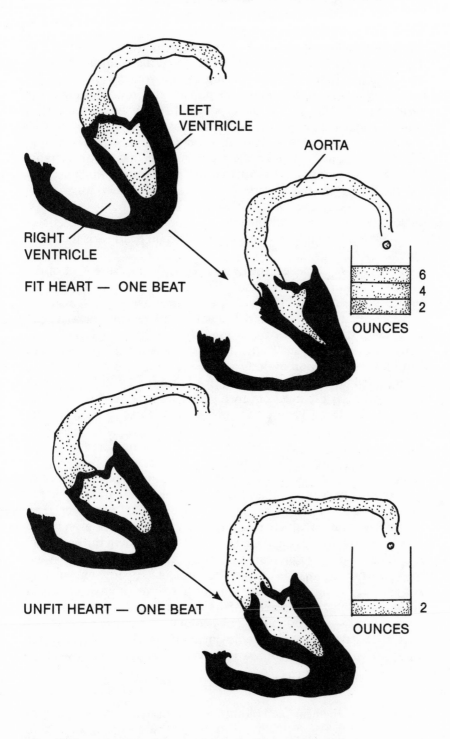

The fit heart pumps more blood with each beat.

the muscles. The amount of blood pumped by the heart in one minute (stroke volume × heart rate) is the *cardiac output.* An unfit person might have a stroke volume of four ounces of blood per beat, so at 190 beats per minute, 48 pints of blood would supply the body each minute. If the same person became fitter, the stroke volume might increase to five ounces of blood per beat, so now 60 pints of blood (the new cardiac output) supplies the body per minute. So we can see how the regular player has a considerably larger reserve pumping capacity that he can call upon when needed. The playful person has a more efficient heart. The heart weighs only about one pound, but during an average lifetime it pumps about 100 million gallons of blood. The combined result of these two effects — more efficient muscles and a more powerful heart — is increased fitness.

There is a way to assess the overall result, by measurement of the oxygen consumption of the body. This is the amount of oxygen the body uses during certain activities, and from it we can calculate the caloric cost of these activities. We could theoretically measure the fuel used instead of the oxygen used to burn it, but oxygen use is easier to measure. Usually this figure is given as the oxygen consumption per kilogram of body weight per minute. When this figure is measured at maximum effort, for instance by collecting and measuring gases breathed out by a person running as fast as he can on a treadmill, we have a measure of *maximum oxygen uptake,* which really tells us how fit the individual is by measuring his greatest capacity for play. Of course, this is a measurement made while playing hard, and you wouldn't do that very often. An extremely sedentary person, who spends much time in bed, might have a maximum oxygen uptake of about 20 milliliters of oxygen per kilogram body weight per minute. At the other end of the scale, an Olympic endurance athlete might have a value of 80, or even more.

To give you a very rough idea of the effect of going through Play Plans A to H during one year, an improvement in maximum oxygen uptake from 35 to 45 might be anticipated for an initially overweight, rather sedentary person, or an improvement in "fitness" of nearly 30 percent. This sort of improvement does not go unnoticed — it is not a mere physiological technicality. It shows itself in less tiredness, more enjoyment of work and play, greater ability to keep up. And fitness is improved by play at *any* age!

CORONARY HEART DISEASE

Diseases of the heart and blood vessels constitute the most important cause of death, disability, distress, sorrow and medical costs in the United States. The leading cause of death in America (1980) was the heart attack; about 1.5 million Americans currently suffer heart attacks each year, of whom about a half-million die.

The underlying cause of the heart attack is a disease of the small coronary arteries that supply blood to the working heart muscle itself. This disease of the artery walls, *atherosclerosis,* is a slow, degenerative process in which the inner lining of the vessels becomes at first roughened and then thickened by accumulations of cholesterol, fibrin and cell debris. Narrowed coronary arteries can easily become blocked by a clot, resulting in sudden, complete withdrawal of blood (with its sustaining oxygen and fuel) to a part of the beating heart (see diagram). This event is a *heart attack,* and results in the death of a portion of the heart muscle. The immediate impact of this can range from almost no effect (a "silent" heart attack) to death. Narrowed coronary arteries are also responsible for angina pectoris, or chest pains during excitement or physical effort. Narrowing and blockage of blood vessels supplying the brain result in stroke.

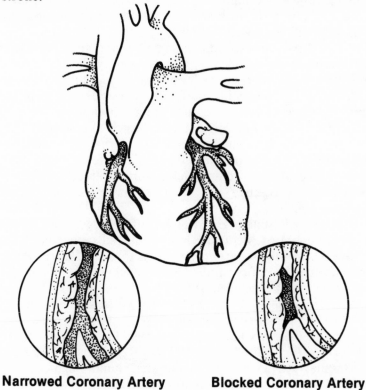

Narrowed Coronary Artery   **Blocked Coronary Artery**

(Courtesy American Heart Association)

Clearly, avoidance of coronary heart disease, and more generally of the underlying artery wall disease, atherosclerosis, would be a great step forward in improving the health and quality of life of vast numbers of Americans. As we saw in Chapter 4, it is not only a question of increasing life span for the average person (and prevention or postponement of coronary heart disease would have some effect on life span). It is also of great significance to prevent, or at least to postpone for as long as possible, the debilitating effects of heart attacks, angina pectoris and related conditions. These ailments, even if they do not kill promptly, put a dent in the ability of millions of us to enjoy the older years that we have in store. There are millions of people who, having experienced one heart attack, will live for many years in fear of another; As Dylan Thomas said,"... poised and brittle, afraid to break, like faded cups and saucers." Let's look at regular play, to see if we can learn anything about avoiding coronary heart disease.

Long-term Studies. A number of studies have been done using the time course approach discussed in Chapter 1. Professor Jeremy Morris and his colleagues followed groups of London double-decker bus drivers and conductors, and found that the occupationally more active conductors, who frequently climbed the stairs to the upper deck, experienced fewer heart attacks than the sedentary drivers. This interesting finding was considered inconclusive because the drivers were found later to have been more obese than the conductors when first hired. Later, Morris also studied a large group of London civil servants, and found that those who were more active in leisure time went on to suffer fewer heart attacks than those who were less active in leisure time. There appeared to be a particularly "protective" effect of the more vigorous types of leisure time activity.

In the United States, Dr. Ralph Paffenbarger, of Stanford University School of Medicine, has conducted pioneering studies that have reached the same conclusions as those of Morris. Paffenbarger and colleagues first studied San Francisco longshoremen for many years, and concluded that those employed in the more physically demanding jobs (cargo handlers) suffered fewer heart attacks than those in less active, supervisory jobs, all other things (that could be measured) being equal. Later, Paffenbarger reported on the six- to 10-year follow-up (1962 to 1972) of nearly 17,000 Harvard alumni aged 35 to 74. Again, the alumni reporting more "habitual and leisure time activity" experienced fewer heart attacks. The following graph shows that the beneficial association was progressive and that "strenuous sports" (including, for instance, running, swimming and tennis) were more influential in reducing risk than were "other activities" (including, for instance, bowling, golf and yard work).

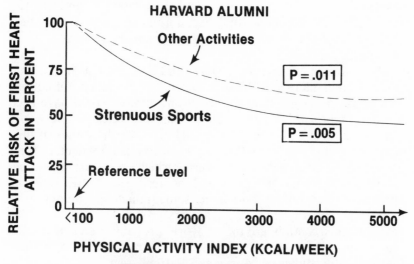

(Courtesy of Ralph Paffenbarger, M.D.)

If we look at the accompanying graph, we see how the amount of activity recorded compares with the play calories expended in the Play Plans of *The California Diet*. The "Reference Level" corresponds to the unplayful state before the program begins, that is, a very sedentary condition. At Play Plan H (300 calories of play per day) we are at the 2100 point on the horizontal axis. At Play Plan J (500 calories of play per day) we are at 3500, which, as you can see, was associated in Paffenbarger's classic study with almost a halving of heart attack rate, especially when the play was in the form of swimming, bicycling, running, tennis and similar activities recommended in this program.

The study also found that a physically active adulthood was associated with lower heart attack rates, whereas athletic involvement at college was not. Other adverse characteristics (smoking, hypertension, history of diabetes and others) considerably increased risk of heart attack; but Paffenbarger showed clearly that for a given adverse characteristic, men with high energy levels had appreciably lower heart attack risk than less energetic college men of the same age (e.g., active smokers did better than sedentary smokers).

In considering their overall results from the study of Harvard men, followed by the time course method for six to 10 years, Paffenbarger and his colleagues concluded:

• If *all* alumni had expended 2000 or more calories per week (Play

Plan H level or above), it is estimated that the number of heart attacks suffered would have been reduced by 26 percent.

• If *all* the men had been physically active (2000 or more calories per week), did not smoke and had normal blood pressure, there would have been only about *half* the number of heart attacks observed.

These are remarkable projections, and it is upon such data that the recommendations of *The California Diet* are based. Of course, we cannot be certain that all these heart attacks would have been avoided or postponed. To establish this with certainty we would have to conduct a vast, expensive trial in which thousands of men were assigned at random either to play or to remain sedentary for a significant portion of their lives, during which time heart attacks occurring in the two groups would be recorded. Under the circumstances, we might anticipate some reluctance among participants to be assigned to the sedentary group. The difficulties inherent in such a study are many: It will probably never be carried out. Meanwhile, we must be guided by the next best information, that from the studies of Morris and Paffenbarger.

Animal Studies. Studies relating to coronary heart disease in animals have the disadvantage of reduced relevance to the human disease, but the distinct advantage of speed. A most intriguing, if preliminary study of exercise in relation to coronary heart disease in monkeys, was reported by Dr. Dieter Kramsch and his colleagues in the *New England Journal of Medicine* in 1981. Groups of young monkeys were assigned to different diets with or without regular exercise comparable to a human jogging for one hour, three times per week. The most interesting comparison involved nine monkeys who were initially on a normal monkey diet for 12 months and then were put on a cholesterol-containing diet (known to promote heart disease in monkeys) for 24 months. These monkeys remained quite sedentary for the entire study. They were compared with nine other monkeys who were also on a normal diet followed by the heart-disease producing diet, but this second group was exercised by running on a treadmill for one hour, three times per week. In other words, one group of monkeys was inactive when it was put on the "atherogenic" diet, and remained inactive for another two years, while the second group was allowed regular play when it was put on the atherogenic diet, and remained playful for another two years.

When examined at the end of the study, the exercised animals were found to have lower resting heart rates (as expected), larger hearts, and coronary arteries — supplying the heart — of greater diameter. The amount of disease of the wall of the coronary arteries was also much less in the exercised monkeys, although both groups had consumed similar amounts of the "bad" diet over two years. The accompanying drawings show magnified cross-sections of the coronary arteries of sedentary and exercised monkeys.

Sedentary   **Exercise**

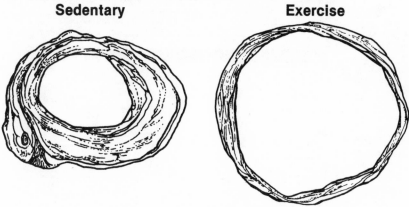

(Courtesy of Dieter Kramsch, M.D.)

Notice that there is less thickening of the inner wall of the artery in the exercised animal, but in addition the diameter (or bore) of the artery is greater in the exerciser. Clearly, the passageway available for flow of blood through these arteries, to supply the monkeys' hearts, is considerably greater for the animal that has played more during its lifetime. The authors summed up their results by pointing out that the benefits derived from moderate exercise in conditions that promoted heart disease (a bad diet) were less atherosclerosis, wider coronary arteries, and a larger heart that functioned at a lower rate.

In fairness, this is a limited, quite preliminary study that urgently needs repetition by other investigators. But it does suggest that regular exercise requiring about three hours per week may help to protect coronary arteries exposed to an atherogenic diet — which is almost certainly the situation faced by the majority of Americans presently. The suggestion that lifelong, regular, moderate play can increase the bore of the coronary arteries is also of great interest in relation to encouraging regular exercise for children.

Research in this area is at a fascinating stage. While awaiting further results, the tentative conclusions for monkeys and men seem clear:

• Improve diet (see Part III)
• Play regularly.

National Heart Disease Trends. If we look at death rates from coronary heart disease in the United States and elsewhere in recent years, we come to three major conclusions:

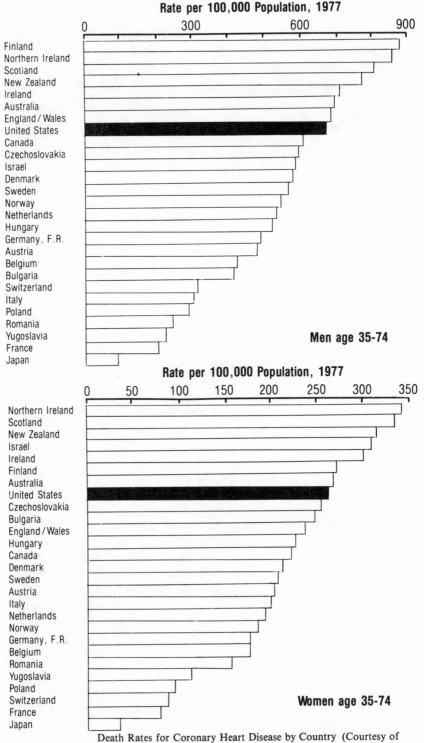

Death Rates for Coronary Heart Disease by Country (Courtesy of
National Heart, Lung and Blood Institute)

• The disease is known in all countries, but there are huge differences in the importance, or the severity, of the disease between nations. This is shown in the accompanying figure, with Finland experiencing almost nine times the death rate of Japan.

• The death rate in a given country is not fixed from year to year. As shown in the graph below(Percent Change in Death Rates), the death rate in the United States from coronary heart disease (and also from stroke) has declined substantially since 1950, although there is still plenty of room for further improvement.

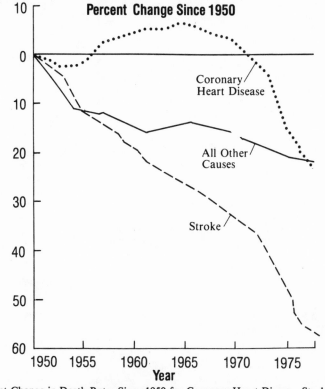

Percent Change in Death Rates Since 1950 for Coronary Heart Disease, Stroke, and All Other Causes , Ages 35-74, United States, 1950-1978.

(Courtesy National Heart, Lung and Blood Institute)

• The *rate* of change in death rate from coronary heart disease is very different among different nations (see pg. 130). In the years 1969 to 1977, some nations have improved death rates, while others have become worse. The United States has the distinction of experiencing the greatest improvement in coronary heart disease death rate, followed by Australia, Canada and Israel.

Clearly, the huge differences and changes in death rates from the United States' major disease must tell us something about what causes the disease and what we might do to hasten its retreat. These

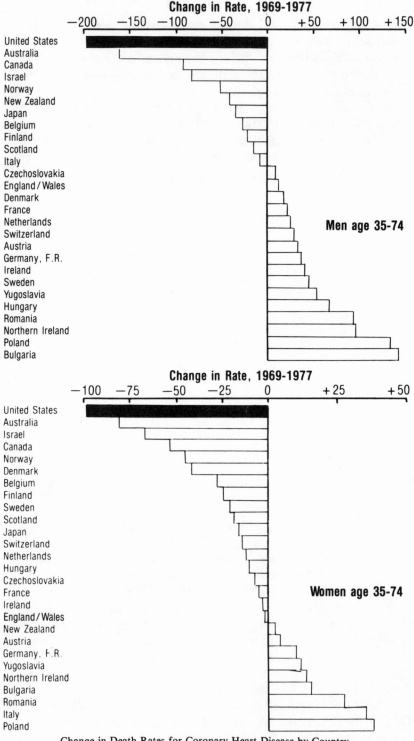

Change in Death Rates for Coronary Heart Disease by Country
(Courtesy National Heart, Lung and Blood Institute.)

figures reflect great "natural experiments," involving millions of deaths. We should interpret them wisely. We do not know all the answers, by any means, presently. But it is now clear that national differences in diet, activity level, obesity, smoking habits and blood pressure levels have a great deal to do with the large differences between countries.

The dramatic decline in the United States coronary heart disease death rates is currently attracting the attention of medical scientists from all over the world. We must have been doing *something* right in the United States recently to account for the decline shown on page 130. Improved treatment of elevated blood pressure, less smoking, national dietary changes, and the "exercise explosion" may all have contributed, as well as improved care of heart attack victims. We don't know how to distribute the credit among these and other factors. But we can at least say that a marked increase in participation in leisure-time play activities — cycling, running, swimming, tennis, racquetball — dating to the late 1960s, is *consistent* with the recent remarkable decline in the United States coronary death rates.

Cholesterol, Lipoproteins and Play. We have seen time course studies that suggest playful people suffer fewer heart attacks, animal studies that suggest a protective role for regular exercise, and that national changes in exercise habits correspond with reduced heart attacks in this country. But how does regular play work its magic? How does it protect against a disease of the inner linings of our arteries?

This is a very active research area, and there are many clues, some of which will be considered later. They include:

• Regular play reduces body fat, which is beneficial for individuals with tendencies toward high blood pressure and diabetes.

• Regular play seems to make the smoking habit superfluous for many people.

• Regular play may bring about mechanical advantages in the heart, such as widened coronary arteries.

• Regular play may relax people.

• Regular play reduces blood pressure levels during work or emotional stress.

• Regular play reduces blood clotting, which might be an advantage to people with already-narrow coronary arteries.

• Regular play changes the cholesterol in the blood in a way that decreases the chances of atherosclerosis, and may actually protect against it.

I will briefly describe recent work on the last clue — the relation of regular play to blood cholesterol levels, since this is a research area that my colleagues and I have been particularly interested in at the Stanford Heart Disease Prevention Program.

Everybody knows that cholesterol has something to do with heart disease: "Too much cholesterol in the blood increases risk of heart disease." This statement is considered today to be essentially true, but taking the subject further, we must consider how cholesterol is carried in the bloodstream. Since cholesterol cannot dissolve in the blood (as salt or sugar does), it must be carried on small particles, called *lipoproteins,* that constantly circulate through our blood vessels, bumping into each other, into red blood cells and into artery walls. The lipoproteins come in three major varieties, of which two carry most of the cholesterol:

PLASMA LIPOPROTEINS

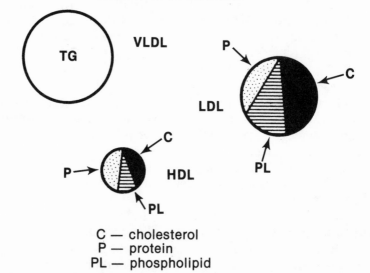

C — cholesterol
P — protein
PL — phospholipid

(From Wood et al., *Ann NY Acad Sci* Vol. 301: 748-763, 1977)

The two types of cholesterol carrier — the larger *low-density lipoproteins,* or LDL, and the smaller *high-density lipoproteins,* or HDL — have very different relationships to the disease atherosclerosis. We've known for years that high LDL levels in the blood are associated with, and almost certainly responsible for coronary artery disease: Individuals with very low levels of LDL particles virtually never have the disease, whereas a few individuals with a genetic disease that produces extremely high blood levels of LDL typically (if untreated) have heart attacks and die before age 20. All of this leads to the belief that high levels of LDL are bad for our arteries.

On the other hand, *low* levels of HDL particles seem to be associated with *increased* risk of coronary heart disease. There is now a great deal of evidence to this effect:

• People who have suffered heart attacks are found to have lower-than-average HDL levels in their blood.

• People with coronary artery disease (as determined from X-ray procedures) have low levels of HDL, and the more extensive the disease, the lower the level.

• Women have *higher* HDL levels than men, and suffer *less* heart disease at comparable ages.

• Animals (for instance the dog and the rat) that are virtually immune from coronary disease, are endowed by nature with high levels of HDL and low levels of LDL.

• Using the time course method, people with low HDL levels have been found to have a greater risk of developing coronary heart disease in future years than people with higher levels.

All of this leads to the conclusion that *low* levels of HDL are bad for our arteries. The best ("least risky") situation is to have a relatively low LDL level and a relatively high HDL level in our bloodstream.

How does all this relate to our play levels? Numerous studies have shown, using the comparison method, that active people tend to have higher HDL levels and lower LDL levels than are found in sedentary people. This is shown in the accompanying figures for groups of middle-aged runners (averaging about 40 miles each week) compared to average men and women of the same age who were relatively sedentary (controls).

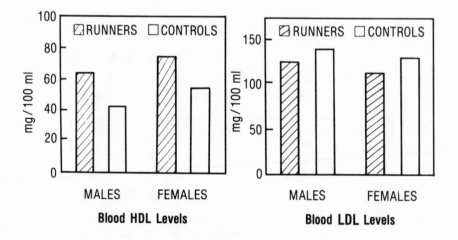

(From Wood et al., *Ann NY Acad Sci* Vol. 301: 748-763, 1977)

In a different approach to the question, 48 sedentary middle-aged men at Stanford University were invited to complete a one-year program of progressive walking, jogging and running. Thirty-three additional men were assigned to remain sedentary. At the end of the year the *change* in HDL level in the blood of the runners were related to the *amount* of running the men achieved during the year, as shown in the following figure:

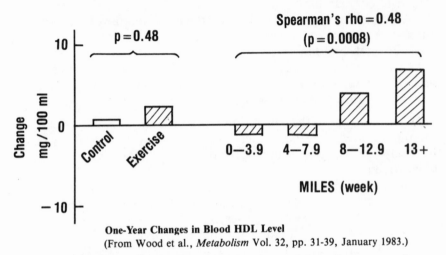

One-Year Changes in Blood HDL Level
(From Wood et al., *Metabolism* Vol. 32, pp. 31-39, January 1983.)

An average running mileage of at least eight miles per week was needed to achieve an increase in HDL compared to the controls. At least four miles per week was required to achieve a decrease in LDL:

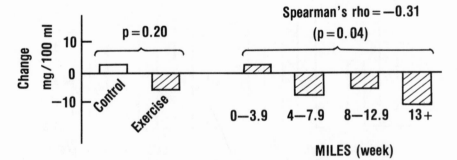

One-Year Changes in Blood LDL Level
(From Wood et al., *Metabolism* Vol. 32, pp. 31-39, January 1983.)

Fourteen of the 48 exercising men agreed to continue for a second year, maintaining an average of 12 miles per week over the entire two-year period. These men showed an increase of 8 percent in their

HDL and a decrease of 6 percent in their LDL over this period. A number of other training studies have shown that increased activity, to the play levels called for in Play Plans H, I and J is accompanied by these changes in HDL and LDL levels in blood, which in turn are associated with lower risk of developing heart disease.

SMOKING, CANCER AND PLAY

It appears that vigorous leisure time exercise is usually accompanied by a rejection of the smoking habit. Years ago, when I was a kid in the Royal Air Force, and 90 percent of my comrades smoked cigarettes, I noticed the one place where there were very few cigarette butts to pick up was at the running track. In studies of dedicated middle-aged runners, we have noticed that virtually no one smokes; however, these players are not lifelong strangers to vice, since a high proportion (39 percent men, 58 percent women) are *ex*-smokers. Many surveys have indicated this trend for the increasingly dedicated player increasingly to reject smoking (perhaps "lose interest in" better describes the evolution of the player to non-smoking, than "reject").

An example of the relative disinterest of older players in the smoking habit is shown in the following survey results of several hundred male members of the Fifty-Plus Runners' Association, in comparison with average men of the same ages:

| | SMOKING RATE (%) | |
AGE	RUNNERS	CONTROLS
50 - 54	5.4	33.9
55 - 59	3.7	24.4
60 - 64	2.6	29.5

Much has been written about the health hazards of smoking. In terms of numbers of people, the hazards of coronary heart disease and heart attack are probably the greatest. A large proportion of all the emphysema and chronic bronchitis in the United States is attributable to cigarette smoking. These two unpleasant diseases alone make the extra years of life given to older people by medical science a doubtful asset for the afflicted. And finally, there are the cancers. Not just lung cancer. Calculations made by Sir Richard Doll and

Dr. Richard Peto, lead to the following conclusions about the contribution of tobacco to cancer deaths in American men in 1978:

CAUSE OF DEATH	NUMBER OF DEATHS		
	OBSERVED	ESTIMATED HAD AMERICAN MEN NOT SMOKED	APPROXIMATE EXCESS ATTRIBUTED TO TOBACCO
Lung cancer	71,006	6,439	64,567
Cancer of mouth, pharynx, larynx or esophagus	14,282	3,584	10,698
Bladder cancer	6,771	2,960	3,811
Cancer of pancreas	11,010	6,585	4,425
Other specified sites	100,799	?	5,000
Unspecified sites	14,469	8,188	6,281
TOTAL	218,337		(43%) 94,782

(Adapted from Doll and Petro, *The Causes of Cancer,* 1981)

According to this estimate by two distinguished epidemiologists, some 43 percent of all male cancer deaths in 1978 could be attributed to smoking. The figure for women is less, since fewer women smoked.

In spite of this depressing insight into determinants of our nation's future health, Americans continue to buy record numbers of cigarettes (628.2 billion in 1980), and the average smoker consumes 11,633 cigarettes each year (or just more than a pack-and-a-half a day). But what groups of Americans have abandoned cigarette smoking? Middle-aged men and women who have become active. So does play help to prevent heart disease and cancer? Judge for yourself.

WEIGHT CONTROL AND FOOD INTAKE

Exercise makes weight loss and weight control easier, which, of course, is the central theme of this book. There are many published studies confirming this contention (see Reference section); and also in America there are millions of once-fat, now-active people willing to testify enthusiastically to the fact.

In the Stanford study mentioned earlier involving 48 initially

sedentary men, we examined the relationship between the amount
of running the men had done individually during the year, the
amount of body fat they had lost or gained, and the change in
calories consumed each day (from records completed by the men).
The changes can be represented like this:

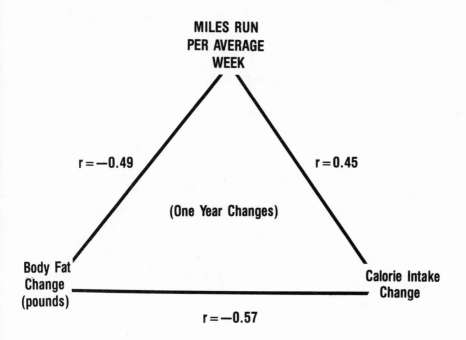

(From Wood et al., *Metabolism* Vol. 32: p. 31-39, 1983)

The "r" values are highly significant correlation coefficients, which
tell us the following:

• The more miles the men ran each week, the more body fat they
lost (r = − 0.49; a *negative* correlation).
• The more miles the men ran each week, the more calories they
reported eating (r = 0.45; a *positive* correlation).
• The greater the *increase* in calorie intake during the year, the
greater the *decrease* in body fat (r = − 0.57; a *negative* correlation).

This last finding tells us that in a one-year play program, the enthusiastic players most successful at losing body fat were also those
who *increased* their food intake the most. So they certainly were not
dieting, were they? Remember that this study was simply to follow

the effects of play: The men were not asked to diet, or indeed to lose weight. They were simply asked to play more, by running regularly, and were observed. If they had dieted by restricting calories, their body fat loss would certainly have been greater. But I think you can see how "eating more but weighing less" can be a reality.

A number of studies have concluded that *maintained* weight loss is more successful when calorie restriction is combined with increased exercise. For instance, Dr. P.M. Stalonas and his colleagues compared a group of overweight women who received instruction only in dieting with another group who were instructed in dieting *and* exercising at a rate of about 400 calories per day (e.g., Play Plan I). After 10 weeks, average weight loss was 23 pounds for the dieters, and 29 pounds for the dieters who also exercised. But at the end of one year, average weight losses for the two groups were 11 pounds (diet only) and 36 pounds (diet and exercise).

So regular play promotes leanness *and* eating more calories, both of which have health benefits. It seems, for instance, that losing weight is ultimately associated with an increase in the HDL cholesterol carrier in the blood, which is believed to be "protective" against heart disease. Exercise often leads to increased calorie intake. As we noticed in Chapter 1, several time course studies have observed that people who developed heart disease reported years earlier eating fewer calories than those in the population who did not die from heart disease:

| | Calories per day reported by: | |
| | Heart Disease | |
Community Studied	Victims	Survivors
U.K., Bank & Busmen	2656	2869
Framingham, MA	2369	2622
Puerto Rico	2223	2395
Honolulu	2149	2319

The average difference in daily calorie consumption for the groups that developed heart disease versus those that did not is about 200 calories per day. This may represent a difference in *play level* (balanced by food intake) of 200 calories per day (as would be provided, for instance, by Play Plan F). We cannot be certain that this 200-calorie difference is because of greater activity among the people who did not develop heart disease, but it seems unlikely that the health advantage was simply attributable to a better appetite.

HIGH BLOOD PRESSURE

According to the American Heart Association, 37 million Americans suffered from high blood pressure in 1980. Sustained high blood pressure can result in damage to three vital organs: the heart, the brain and the kidneys. Hypertension (high blood pressure) is thus an enormous public health challenge.

How does hypertension relate to exercise? First, we should know that blood pressure is usually measured in the resting state (the doctor says, "Sit quietly for a few minutes, and then I'll take your blood pressure."). The resting state, quiescent and relaxed, has long been the standard circumstance for measurement of "blood pressure." But an increase in blood pressure is a normal, indeed an essential reaction to exercise. To minimize risk of damage to the heart (heart attack), the brain (stroke) or the kidneys (kidney failure), it is desirable to have a relatively low resting blood pressure, and also to avoid very high blood pressure levels during the working, worry-filled day.

Regular play activities help in the following ways:

• Exercise leads to lower body weight and control of obesity. Reduction of obesity is the first step in treating hypertension, since weight loss is almost always accompanied by a reduction of resting blood pressure.

• Many studies have shown that the blood pressure resulting from exercise (for instance, running on a treadmill at six miles per hour) is *reduced* as a result of training. In other words, the physically fit, playful individual can sustain *lower* blood pressure while working out than a sedentary individual who is not accustomed to such activity. This is a very important benefit of regular play that tends to be overlooked, since blood pressure is so frequentlly measured only in the resting state. But take the case of two people, one active, the other sedentary. Perhaps both have the same "resting" blood pressure, 125/87 mm of mercury. But if both individuals are obliged to run for a bus, the sedentary person's blood pressure may rise to 190/100, whereas the fit person's blood pressure rises to only 160/90. It is very possible that the peaks of blood pressure reached are very significant with respect to organ damage. We shall learn much more about this in future research; meanwhile, we do know that regular play tends to reduce these blood pressure peaks.

• The time course studies of Morris and Paffenbarger, which have been referred to earlier, both suggest that regular exercise is valuable in heading off hypertension, particularly in younger people who are overweight. It is less clear that regular play influences *resting* blood pressure in older people, or in people who are not overweight.

DIABETES

Diabetes appears most frequently in middle-aged people who are overweight. Adult-onset (non-insulin requiring) diabetics are improved, and often returned to a non-diabetic status, by weight loss. For this reason moderate exercise, to assist in weight control, is valuable for diabetics. Diabetes can sharply increase risk of heart attack.

The hormone, insulin, produced by the pancreas, has the function of arranging the transfer of blood glucose (from the diet) into the tissues that use it. If the system does not work, the tissues remain low in glucose, and sugar piles up in the blood and spills over into the urine. This is diabetes. Only in one type of diabetics, who are dependent on regular injections of insulin, is insulin actually absent or in short supply. Most adult diabetics are overweight and have plenty of insulin; the problem is that their tissues have become insensitive to the insulin they do have. This is where exercise comes in: Exercise increases tissue sensitivity to insulin, making insulin "go further." A diabetic who does inject with insulin must take care to adjust his insulin dose to his exercise level, since less insulin is needed when exercising.

BONES AND JOINTS

Regular activity, especially in middle age and beyond, is of particular interest in relation to two important diseases: arthritis and osteoporosis.

Osteoporosis is a progressive disease in which minerals, particularly calcium, are lost from the bones faster than they are replaced. So the bones slowly become more porous and brittle. Older women are particularly prone to fractures resulting from bones weakened by osteoporosis. About one million fractures are experienced each year by American women age 45 or older; of these, 700,000 are incurred by women with osteoporosis. This is a serious condition, since about 50 percent of elderly women who incur femoral neck fractures die within one year. Increased dietary calcium and estrogen replacement are standard treatments for osteoporosis. However, institution of regular exercise in elderly women may be beneficial in stimulating retention of minerals by bones. An active life, with regular exercise, probably brings a woman to older age with stronger bones and muscles than would result from years of sedentary living. And it has been shown that active people have denser bones than sedentary people.

Arthritis is an extremely disabling disease of middle and old age. Coronary heart disease is America's major killer, but arthritis is

America's major disabler. The relation of regular exercise to arthritis — both as a preventive and as a treatment — is an important research area, particularly in view of the shift of America's population to older age groups, and of the increasing acceptance of regular play as an important part of life. This is a research area where the verdict — either for or against regular exercise — is not clear yet. However, a few observations are defensible.

• Both very sedentary and very active people can develop osteoarthritis.
  • Damage to joints may promote arthritis.
  • Regular use of joints eases stiffness due to arthritis.
  • Limited studies on lifelong runners and skiers indicate "average" degrees of osteoarthritis in hip joints.

CONSTIPATION

Constipation has been held responsible for a number of serious conditions — from diverticulosis to colon cancer — by some authorities. Clearly, we are better off without this "disease of civilization." Inclusion of adequate fiber in the diet, to provide "bulk" (see Chapter 10) is part of the solution to the problem. Very active people also appear to be afflicted by constipation less often. Perhaps this is because of the mechanical action of walking, bicycling and running. Another interesting explanation is that since very active people eat more, more food residues enter the colon, giving this organ more material to work on, thus reducing constipation. Certainly, the inactive person with a low-calorie, low-residue diet is a prime candidate for constipation.

A recent survey of several hundred members of the Fifty-Plus Runners' Association indicated that constipation is a relatively rare affliction among this very playful group.

SEX

Whether or not regular exercise improves our sex life cannot be judged on the basis of existing scientific studies. The paucity of high-quality (and hence, expensive-to-acquire) information to tell us whether or not regular exercise makes for better sex, is no cause for surprise, since public money could not reasonably be spent on such a flippant (although widely interesting) subject. Pending funding of research projects in this area, we might say that regular exercise is sexually advantageous because:

• It leads to feelings of confidence in one's body — a prerequisite for good sex. It promotes improved "self-esteem."

• It leads to a slim figure, generally held in our society to be sexually desirable.

• It leads to increased fitness and health, which must be the foundation of all physical endeavors.

THE MIND

As with the previous topic, the volume of good research on the influence of exercise on the mind is not overwhelming. But, since this is a subject of great interest to all who exercise regularly, there is no shortage of anecdotes and opinions.

• There is a remarkably widespread and consistent belief on the part of regular exercisers that their play makes them "feel better." Exercisers report that they "feel worse" when they don't exercise! We don't know why this very desirable and reinforcing effect of exercise occurs. It may be related to increased production of "brain opiates," the endorphins (the morphine within), which increase in concentration in the blood during vigorous exercise. While we are busy finding out why regular play has this widely reported effect, it is nice to know that there is something that is cheap, accessible and relatively non-addictive that can provide what humanity desires: to feel better.

• There is preliminary evidence that an exercise program may change Type A behavior (which has been shown to increase risk of heart attack) in a beneficial way. This topic is certainly worthy of further research in this time-urgent, impatient world.

• Several studies, including pioneer work by Dr. Thaddeus Kostrubala, suggest that group running may be a useful therapy for people with certain mental conditions, notably depression. In some circumstances exercise has proved to be at least as effective as traditional drug treatments, without the sometimes serious side effects.

• In suitable circumstances, physical achievements can have enormous curative and restorative powers for people who have encountered adversity. One example: A few years ago I completed the Boston Marathon with some members of Dr. Terence Kavanagh's team of post-heart-attack marathon runners, with their distinctive "mended heart" T-shirts, to tumultuous applause from the Boston crowds. The boost to morale for men who had only recently entertained profound doubts about their future physical capabilities, has to be experienced to be believed. This is a therapy not available from a medical center or pharmacy.

PART THREE: INGREDIENTS FOR A HEALTHY DIET

9. Carbohydrates, Fat, Protein

At this point we have looked at the features of a good weight-loss program, and considered the important place that regular play should have in our lives. One task remains: to consider how best to construct our diets over the years. The concern is not so much the quantity of food we eat, which should reflect our play level, but what sort of food we should eat. The next three chapters will address this complex area.

THE AMERICAN FOOD SUPPLY

Decisions about what to eat were much easier at earlier stages of our evolutionary history. When the diet of many North Americans consisted largely of ground acorns, I suppose the major food problem was to ensure a good supply of acorns. Contrast the dilemma of the modern North American. He or she ventures out from a home already stocked with many food items, and proceeds down the street to the supermarket, which contains a bewildering array of foods. From the thousands of different items, perhaps 30 will be selected by some mechanism that is difficult to describe — or to guide. Some choices are astonishingly sophisticated by historical standards: Which of three competing brands of olives stuffed with pimentos should I purchase? Perhaps it's to the liquor store next, with its thousands of brands of alcoholic beverages: which of 30 Scotch whiskeys? Which of a hundred beers? And then home again, via the bookstore, which has 30 magazines offering advice on what to eat this week, 50 cookbooks telling how to cook it, and a hundred diet books offering help in resisting all this temptation, and giving instructions on how to "eat less." Under these circumstances, it is hardly surprising that our population, although remarkably well nourished in many respects, is rather confused about many fundamental nutritional issues, and in fact consumes widely divergent ɑiets. Women traditionally have a big responsibility here, since more often than not they make the choices that determine the nature of the family's food intake over many years.

Who Eats What and When?

A major scientific task is the assessment of what a population, such as that of the United States, is actually eating. Once we know what are the current eating patterns, we can follow the effects of any attempts that may be made to improve those patterns. Since there is so much diversity in food selection, we need to know the answers for specific groups: old and young, male and female, pregnant and non-pregnant women, prosperous and poor, and by geographical region. Large, representative samples must be studied, usually by asking people to recall in detail what they ate in the past 24 hours, or by asking them to complete personal food records for a number of days. But there are many problems: People are forgetful; often they never knew what they were eating or didn't notice; some people are sensitive about disclosing their true alcohol intake; and estimates of portion sizes vary considerably. All of this information has to be converted into major nutrients (fat, protein, carbohydrate, specific vitamins); a list of 97 foods eaten in a week is of little use without this breakdown. So data on the composition of thousands of foods have to be available. There are other approaches. We could measure the total amount of food entering U.S. households and restaurants and divide by the size of the population. But this would give a false, high per capita consumption level, because there is a great deal of food waste. Random sampling of garbage cans has even been done in attempts to measure average household food waste.

I have spent time on this diet assessment issue because it is very important to know what people eat (if eating relates to health, as it certainly does); and also because it is complex, expensive and inconvenient to find out in a satisfactorily scientific manner. This all results from the complexity of our modern diets. If we ate nothing but acorns, it would be so simple!

In spite of the many problems, several good studies of America's food intake have been conducted in recent years, by the Health and Nutrition Examination Survey (HANES) and the Lipid Research Clinics (LRC) prevalence surveys, to name two. Comments in the next three chapters on "what people eat" are based on the findings of such surveys, rather than on general impressions.

Who Should Eat What? The next big question is what people *should* eat. Asking and attempting to answer this question has assumed the proportions of a major industry today. A rapid and admittedly inexpensive mechanism for providing answers is fiat, as in: "Thou shalt eat pineapple." In spite of the scientific shortcomings of this approach, there is no question that many nutritional choices are prompted simply because an individual has asserted (often without benefit of scientific evidence) that a given food is good, or bad. The foods featured in *The California Diet* were selected on the basis of current scientific consensus, so far as this can be determined. After all, we all pay taxes to have scientists conduct expensive studies relating to food choices — we may as well benefit from this investment.

The available scientific information about food selection comes from three major sources:

• Animal studies. Results from animal studies can be obtained faster and cheaper, and information obtained is often much more detailed, compared to human studies. Of course, lack of relevance to the human condition can be a severe limitation. Nonetheless, historically this method has contributed a great deal.

• Metabolic ward studies. Human volunteers are studied in a controlled, scientific setting. Metabolic ward studies are precise, but extremely expensive.

• Population studies. Time course studies of dietary habits in relation to health and disease in large populations can be illuminating. The work is expensive and lengthy — a study of 10 or more years is not unusual. It is extremely difficult to influence food intake habits significantly in large populations, as can be done readily in animal and metabolic ward studies. Such large-scale public education projects will no doubt become more frequent. But often "natural experiments" have been available for study, with valuable conclusions. For instance, health of a population with a certain diet (e.g., the Japanese) can be compared with that of a population with a very different diet (e.g., the U.S. population). Again, World War II resulted in dramatic changes in the dietary intake of entire populations (e.g., Germany), with accompanying health changes that have been followed.

The total nutritional information obtained from these three methods is enormous, and yet much more needs to be learned. Space does not permit a consideration of individual studies (consult Reference section for major reviews), but the knowledge available has been distilled into several key reports that will be referred to in chapters 9, 10 and 11, and that have been considered in constructing the menu plans and foods recommended in *The California Diet*.

The most important reports are:

Dietary Goals for the United States (2nd edition). Select Committee on Nutrition and Human Needs (1977).

Nutrition and Your Health. Dietary Guidelines for Americans. U.S. Department of Agriculture and U.S. Department of Health, Education and Welfare (1980).

Healthy People. The Surgeon General's Report on Health Promotion and Disease Prevention. Public Health Service, U.S. Department of Health, Education and Welfare (1979).

Recommended Dietary Allowances (9th edition). The National Research Council (1980).

Diet and Coronary Heart Disease. American Heart Association (1978).

Arteriosclerosis 1981. Report of the Working Group on Arteriosclerosis of the National Heart, Lung and Blood Institute. U.S. Department of Health and Human Services (1981).

The Causes of Cancer. Richard Doll and Richard Peto. Oxford University Press (1981).

THE MAJOR NUTRIENTS: CARBOHYDRATE, FAT AND PROTEIN

In spite of the diversity of diets consumed throughout the world, there are six components that are present in virtually all diets. Some have energy value (they can provide fuel) and others do not:

	Calories per gram
Carbohydrate	4
Fat	9
Protein	4
Vitamins	0
Minerals	0
Water	0

All of these components are essential to healthy life, although it is possible to exist on a diet that is extremely low in fat. Water, the solvent for the body's chemical reactions, is the most essential item. In a matter of hours under extremely hot conditions, the body can become critically short of water. Vitamins and minerals are essential, but provide no calories. They will be considered in Chapter 10.

There is one other dietary component that provides part (sometimes a significant part) of the calorie intake for many people — alcohol. One gram (about one-thirtieth of an ounce) of pure alcohol produces seven calories when metabolized. This rather unique and extremely variable component of the diet will be discussed in Chapter 11.

We will discuss in this chapter the desirable amounts and proportions of the three major calorie-providing components of the diet: carbohydrate, fat and protein. One pointer to the "best" distribution of these three components comes from the Recommended Dietary Allowances (RDA). These recommendations have been published since 1943 at approximately five-year intervals by the Committee on Dietary Allowances, and are defined as follows:

Recommended Dietary Allowances (RDA) are the levels of intake of essential nutrients considered, in the judgment of the Committee on Dietary Allowances of the Food and Nutrition Board on the basis of available scientific knowledge, to be adequate to meet the known nutritional needs of practically all healthy persons.

The RDAs have been published (most recently, in 1980) for vitamins (fat-soluble and water-soluble) and minerals, and for protein. Desirable intakes for fat and carbohydrate, although of great interest in relation to health, are not the subject of RDAs. However, there is a Recommended Dietary Allowance for total protein, since some protein components are clearly essential. A good starting point, then, is to ensure that protein content of the diet is adequate. Separate RDAs are published for infants and children, for males and for females of various ages, and for pregnant and lactating women.

The calorie plans (pages 203-230) given in *The California Diet* meet RDAs for adult men and women for virtually all nutrients at all calorie levels. This is not true for many popular weight-loss diets; and for some the content of nutrients is not disclosed, and has probably not been calculated.

Carbohydrates

There are three major types of dietary carbohydrate:

- Sugars — simple carbohydrates
- Starches — complex carbohydrates
- Fiber — non-digestible carbohydrate and carbohydrate-like components of food.

All three should be considered in planning a well-constructed diet.

In many parts of the world the starches, or complex carbohydrates, are the major energy source in the diet. The starch of rice, soy, potato, wheat and corn propels Nepalese endlessly up steep trails in the Himalayas and provides the power for millions of Chinese to pedal their bicycles. Starch provides 70 to 80 percent or more of total calories for many of the world's people. If they are very active — for instance Nepalese porters — they must eat large amounts of starch, such as rice, since starches are not calorie-dense foods. In the United States, the current diet contains on average about 22 percent of calories as complex carbohydrates, which is quite low by world standards. This has not always been so. It is estimated that in 1909 43 percent of U.S. calories came from starches. It is fascinating to reflect that so many of the spectacular "man made" achievements of the past — from construction of the Egyptian pyramids to building our country's first transcontinental railway — have been powered by starch.

The vast majority of these starch eaters, past and present, have been lean. We often hear dieters decline to eat potatoes (largely starch), because they're "fattening." Anything is fattening if one is sufficiently inactive! But starches certainly do not deserve the label "fattening." It is also noteworthy that populations on a high-starch diet (many Japanese and Indians) have very low levels of coronary heart disease. Conversely, populations on a high-fat diet (Finland and the United States) have high rates of heart disease. Starches are exclusively *vegetable,* so they are often associated with nutritious components (vitamins and minerals), but are free of the exclusively animal product, *cholesterol.* It appears, then, that a diet reasonably high in complex carbohydrates has a good deal to be said for it from a health standpoint.

Sugars, which are simple carbohydrates, occur naturally in fruits, milk and honey, among other sources. Complex carbohydrates are converted to simple sugars during digestion, and circulate in the bloodstream as glucose. During the 20th century, developed countries have incorporated more simple sugars into their diet, by growing sugar cane and sugar beet on a large scale, and making refined sugar (sucrose) from it to add to foods. They have also chemically processed starches (as occurs in digestion) to produce simple sugars, as in corn syrup. A taste for sweetness has been cultivated as a result of this. In the current U.S. diet, refined and processed sugar contributes about 18 percent to total calories, while naturally occurring sugars (particularly in fruit and milk) contribute about 6 percent. Added to the 22 percent complex carbohydrates, the U.S. diet currently derives about 46 percent of total calories from carbohydrates of all types.

There is considerable debate about the appropriate proportion of simple sugars — and especially of ordinary "sugar" or sucrose — in the well-constructed diet. This issue will be looked at in more detail in Chapter 11.

The last category of carbohydrate is fiber. This is non-digestible, and so makes no contribution to dietary calories. Fiber is vegetable in origin, and occurs in fruits, vegetables and grains. Good examples are apples and whole wheat bread. Apple juice and white bread have had the fiber removed. Fiber provides "bulk" in the diet, and clearly facilitates the process of elimination. Many nutrition experts believe that fiber has other valuable functions in relation to our health, as is discussed in Chapter 11.

Fat

Fat has a special place in animal and plant biology by virtue of its high *caloric density*. To put this another way, fat packs a great deal of energy into relatively little weight. And so fat occurs as the prime form of energy storage in animals (e.g., fat, hibernating bears and overweight, sedentary people) and plants (e.g., the avocado and the peanut, both rich in fat). Since fats and oils (which are simply liquid fats) are so commonly used for energy storage in both animals and plants, they occur frequently in our food supply. The human body also uses this method of storing surplus energy for a time of need. If a person eats more fat than he or she needs immediately, the excess is stored in the "adipose tissue" as fat. But if the person eats more starch than he or she needs, this also is converted to fat and stored, so it is possible to become very fat on a low-fat diet. It is the very compact nature of fat that allowed our ancestors of thousands of years ago to survive many hard winters. The same *weight* of less calorie-dense carbohydrate, stored in the body, simply would not have provided enough fuel.

Now the high caloric density of fat is backfiring on us in the Western world. Where calories are generally abundant, an acquired liking for the texture and taste of fat has made it all too easy for the sedentary person to eat too much fat. It is not so much a problem of eating too many calories (as we have seen in Part I), but rather of eating too high a *proportion* of fat in the diet. The current U.S. diet includes about 42 percent of calories from fat.

There are two other major points related to fat consumption. First, much of America's fat is of animal origin: beef, lamb, pork, chicken, butter, eggs. All of these sources contain cholesterol, and it is in reality a "high-fat, high-cholesterol diet." (This does not have to be true elsewhere. For instance, Eskimos, in some areas, eat a diet rich in fish and seal meat, which provides a high-fat but relatively low-cholesterol diet). *Vegetable fats and oils do not contain cholesterol.*

The second point is that there are different kinds of fat. Animal fats tend to contain higher proportions of the harder, *saturated* fats.

Vegetable oils tend to contain higher proportions of the liquid, *polyunsaturated* fats. Both animal and vegetable oils and fats often contain considerable amounts of the intermediate *monounsatuated* fats. Olive oil and avocados, for instance, are very rich in monoun-saturated fats. The ratio of polyunsaturated to saturated fats in a fat or oil is known as the "P/S ratio," and this value is given for each menu plan in this program.

Certain dietary polyunsaturated fats are vital to human health — they are "essential," and cannot be made in the body, like vitamins, and so must be obtained from the diet. Linoleic acid usually serves this function in human diets. A *minimum* of 2 percent of total calories from linoleic acid (contained, among other sources, in corn oil and safflower oil) is recommended. In fact, the current U.S. diet provides, on average, about 6 percent of calories from linoleic acid, so this particular requirement is already well taken care of for most Americans.

These different types of fat also appear to have an influence on health via their effect on blood levels of the cholesterol carrier, LDL (low density lipoprotein) (see page 132). Diets rich in saturated fat tend to increase levels of LDL, which is implicated in the process leading to coronary heart disease. On the other hand, diets relatively rich in polyunsaturated fats tend to reduce LDL levels. Monoun-saturated fats are "neutral" in their effect on LDL. The whole sub-ject of the influence of different types of fat upon risk of coronary heart disease, and so on health, has been vigorously debated for many years, and has been complicated by the related issue of dietary cholesterol. As we shall see, the present consensus is to move to lower levels of intake of *total* fat, but within this lower level to decrease saturated fat and increase polyunsaturated fat intake (an increase in P/S ratio). This translates into a move toward vegetable fat sources (which has already occurred to some extent in the United States). Accompanying a move toward vegetable fat sources, there will be a tendency to eat less cholesterol (e.g. eggs, dairy products, meat), which is also generally seen as desirable. Again, it seems that U.S. dietary cholesterol intake has also dropped in recent years. These clear, but not yet large changes in the nation's dietary intake may be in part responsible for the accompanying decline in U.S. death rate from coronary heart disease, noted in Chapter 8.

In addition to the fairly clear indictment against high-fat (especially high saturated fat) diets by reason of their association with high rates of heart disease, there is increasing evidence — and concern — relating high-fat consumption with high rates of certain cancers. For instance, death rates from breast cancer in countries such as Thailand and Japan, where daily fat intake is less than 45 grams per day, are less than 5 per 100,000 population, whereas in

New Zealand and Denmark, with daily fat intakes of more than 150 grams per day, death rates are about 25 per 100,000 — five times higher. There is also a strong correlation between meat consumption and colon cancer: For instance, Nigeria and Japan (negligible meat eaters) have very low rates, whereas the United States and New Zealand (champion meat eaters) have very high rates.

These striking associations between high-fat and meat intakes and high rates of certain cancers cannot be taken as absolute proof that the "affluent" diet causes these cancers. There are other biological reasons to suggest a mechanism whereby cause and effect could operate. Meanwhile, the consensus (but no means the *only* view) is that a move of the U.S. national diet toward a *lower* fat content would be desirable.

Protein

Proteins are building blocks for much of the vital structure of the body, and make up the enzymes that allow it to operate. Body proteins are in a constant state of flux, and need to be replaced regularly. The complex protein molecule is assembled in the cells, but a variety of *amino acids* must be available to the cells for this to happen. Of the 20 or so amino acids, nine cannot be made by the human body, yet are *essential.* They must be supplied in the diet.

With this in mind, the RDA for protein has been set at 56 grams per day for adult men and 44 grams per day for adult women, with an *additional* 30 grams per day recommended for pregnant women and 20 grams per day for lactating women. Generally, the American population is well above these allowances. For instance, the Lipid Research Clinics survey (1971-74) recorded an average daily protein intake in surveys of several thousand men and women of 102 grams per day for men and 70 grams for women, which amounted to 15 to 16 percent of total calories from protein. Protein deficiency is thus a very unusual problem in the United States, although people who adopt vegetarian diets should be careful to ensure that their protein supply is adequate in *quality,* i.e., adequate amounts of the essential amino acids are present. For a good explanation of this subject, see *Diet for a Small Planet* (Reference section).

A deficiency of protein is unfortunately a feature of the diets of millions of the world's less fortunate, and leads to the disease kwashiorkor, a word of African origin. In comparison, the United States, with up to 16 percent of total calories from protein, is relatively profligate with this nutrient. The answer to the question "Should I take protein supplements?" is therefore "No" in almost all American cases. Even for athletes performing hard muscular work, and "building muscle," there is no evidence that additional protein is helpful above the levels normally taken in with their increased total food intake.

Since Americans eat more protein than they need for replacement of tissues, what happens to the excess? The nitrogen part of protein is removed from the body (as urea, in the urine) and the remainder is either used for fuel (which makes protein a supplementary source of energy, after carbohydrate and fat), or is converted to carbohydrate or fat. Too many calories, in the form of excess protein, can contribute to excess stored fat, just as can a superfluity of fat or carbohydrate in the diet. Although the body can deal well with a moderate excess of protein above replacement needs, very high protein diets (as in some weight-loss programs) are undesirable or even dangerous, as discussed in Chapter 1.

WHAT THE UNITED STATES POPULATION EATS

Having discussed some of the evidence suggesting what a well-constructed diet should look like, let's return briefly to what the United States population actually eats. The survey data available to us vary, reflecting the difficulty of making these measurements, the period of time covered by the surveys (dietary habits are changing!) and whether or not alcohol — a significant source of calories — is included. The report *Dietary Goals for the United States* used a breakdown (opposite page) of calorie sources for the average adult male and female, excluding alcoholic beverages.

The Lipid Research Clinic surveys produced results that are reasonably similar.

In relation to our discussion of a well-constructed diet, the most notable features of this "typical American diet" — which will be close to the diet of the typical *overweight* American — are these:

• Fat (42 percent calories) is a high proportion of total calories.

• Saturated fats (16 percent) and monounsaturated fats (19 percent) are high proportions of total fat, and polyunsaturated fat (7 percent) is rather a low proportion.

• Protein (12 percent) is quite adequately represented in the diet.

• Complex carbohydrates (starches), at 22 percent of total calories, are very low.

• Refined and processed sugars (18 percent) are very high.

Alcohol intake adds, on average, about 200 calories per day to the diet of adult Americans. But since some Americans don't drink, and others drink heavily, the influence of alcohol on construction of an individual's diet varies. For a considerable number of Americans, alcohol provides 10 to 20 percent of total calories or

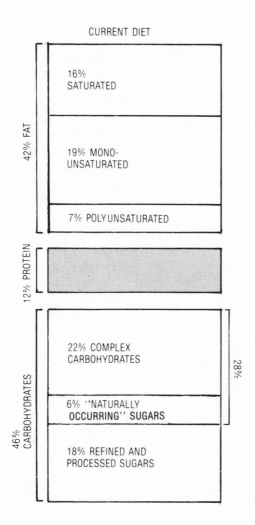

CURRENT DIET

42% FAT

16% SATURATED

19% MONO-UNSATURATED

7% POLYUNSATURATED

12% PROTEIN

46% CARBOHYDRATES

22% COMPLEX CARBOHYDRATES

28%

6% "NATURALLY OCCURRING" SUGARS

18% REFINED AND PROCESSED SUGARS

more on a very regular basis. These calories are usually "empty," meaning that they are not accompanied by vitamins and minerals.

We must also remember that the American diet is changing: Large changes have occurred in the past 70 years, and quite significant changes in the past 10 years. In addition, nationwide surveys take several years to organize, conduct, analyze and publish, and so rapidly become outdated. Some very recent trends are not taken into account by the survey data used in *Dietary Goals for the United States,* which was published in 1974. Since that time there has been a recession, which may influence eating patterns. There is an impression, difficult to document, that today more people are embracing vegetarianism. Diets such as that proclaimed by Nathan Pritikin (a food selection bordering on vegetarianism, with a very low total fat content) have become familiar to many people, but the true adherence to such diets is difficult to assess. Some other major U.S. changes in recent years may have an associated influence on people's food choices. For instance, both comparison studies and time course studies conducted by our group at Stanford Heart Disease Prevention Program suggest that people who become very active, for instance by taking up running, tend not only to eat more, but also to select a somewhat higher carbohydrate, lower fat diet. If this is confirmed, you might expect the U.S. "exercise explosion" to have made an impact on national food choices, which in turn could eventually affect the nation's health.

Recommendations

Dietary Goals for the United States recommends the following changes in average intake of fat, carbohydrate and protein for adults:

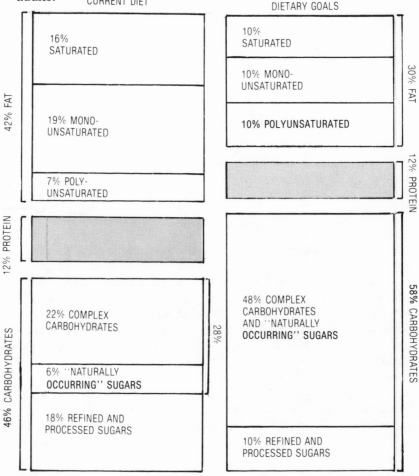

• Total fat to be reduced from the present 42 percent to 30 percent of total calories.

• Proportions of saturated, monounsaturated and polyunsaturated fats to be adjusted to 10 percent each of total calories.

• Protein to be 12 percent of total calories.

• Total carbohydrate to be increased from 46 percent to 58 percent of total calories; of which 48 percent of calories should be from complex plus naturally occurring sugars, and 10 percent from refined and processed sugars.

The Dietary Guidelines for Americans, which rephrases the Dietary Goals in more familiar nutritional terms, calls for the following changes in American eating habits:

• Eat a variety of foods.
• Avoid too much fat, saturated fat and cholesterol.
• Eat foods with adequate starch and fiber.
• Avoid too much sugar.

The Recommended Dietary Allowance calls for 56 grams of protein per day for adult males, 44 grams for adult females.

THE WELL-CONSTRUCTED DIET

The California Diet and Exercise Program has five calorie plans (1200, 1600, 2000, 2400, 2800 calories; pp. 203-230). At the end of each plan is the Nutritional Content, listing the average daily intake of nutrients provided by that plan. For instance, the fat, carbohydrate and protein part of the 2400 Calorie Plan (page 219) looks like this:

2400 CALORIE PLAN

NUTRITIONAL CONTENT

(AVERAGE DAILY INTAKE OVER SEVEN DAYS OF PLAN)

CALORIES	2375
PROTEIN (grams)	106
TOTAL FAT (grams)	74
TOTAL CARBOHYDRATES (grams)	322
% PROTEIN CALORIES	18
% FAT CALORIES	28
% CARBOHYDRATE CALORIES	54
POLYUNSATURATED/SATURATED FAT (P/S) RATIO	1.16
REFINED SUGAR (grams)	7
NATURAL SIMPLE SUGARS (grams)	146
STARCH (grams)	160

CHOLESTEROL (milligrams)	312
CALCIUM (milligrams)	1206
PHOSPHORUS (milligrams)	1781
MAGNESIUM (milligrams)	558
IRON (milligrams)	22
ZINC (milligrams)	18
VITAMIN A (International units)	12,637
THIAMINE (milligrams)	2.0
RIBOFLAVIN (milligrams)	2.7
NIACIN (milligrams)	27
VITAMIN C (milligrams)	186
VITAMIN B_6 (milligrams)	3.1
FOLACIN (micrograms)	440

The plan provides about 106 grams of protein (18 percent of total calories), which is well above the RDA for adult men of 56 grams per day, and for pregnant females of 74 grams per day. All calorie plans exceed these RDAs. Fat calories provide 28 percent of the total calories, which is close to the 30 percent level recommended in the U.S. Dietary Goals. Fat calories for all calorie plans are below 30 percent of total calories. The P/S ratio for the 2400 Calorie Plan is 1.16. P/S ratios for all plans are close to the 1.0 ratio called for in the U.S. Dietary Goals. Refined sugar is seven grams for the 2400 Calorie Plan — and all plans have low levels of refined sugar, as the U.S. Dietary Goals recommend. Total carbohydrates make up 54 percent of total calories — close to the 58 percent figure recommended in the U.S. Dietary Goals.

In addition, all the calorie plans are in general conformity with the U.S. Dietary Guidelines: They feature a variety of foods, avoid too much fat, saturated fat and cholesterol, contain adequate starch and fiber, and avoid too much sugar.

In short, *The California Diet* features meal plans that not only provide appropriate calorie levels, but also conform to the latest scientific advice on fat, carbohydrate and protein content.

10. Vitamins, Minerals, Fiber

Vitamins and minerals (the micronutrients) and fiber occupy a special position in the diet: They are important for maintenance of health, but make no contribution to energy supply.

VITAMINS

Vitamins are a class of compounds that are essential to human life, provide no energy (unlike essential amino acids) and cannot be made by the body; they must be provided by the diet.

A substance may be a vitamin for one animal species, but not for another. For instance, cholesterol, which is readily made by the human body, is a vitamin for the cockroach, since this insect cannot make cholesterol, and without it the creature eventually dies.

Vitamins are divided into two major classes: 1) fat-soluble vitamins (dissolve in fat preferentially) and 2) water-soluble vitamins (dissolve in water preferentially).

The vitamins have different functions in the body; some have multiple functions. A number of substances, some ill-defined, have been promoted as vitamins, for which there is inadequate scientific evidence of "essentialness." "Vitamin B_{15}" and "Vitamin B_{17}" (laetrile) are examples.

A description of the function of all vitamins is out of place here. But the major vitamins considered in constructing the diets in this program are as follows (with the maximum adult male RDA in usual units):

Fat-Soluble Vitamins
Vitamin A   (5000 International Units)

Water-Soluble Vitamins
Thiamine   (1.4 milligrams)
Riboflavin   (1.6 milligrams)

Niacin	(18 milligrams)
Vitamin C	(60 milligrams)
Vitamin B$_6$	(2.2 milligrams)
Folacin	(400 micrograms)

The RDAs are higher for pregnant or lactating women.

The vitamin section of the nutritional content for the 2400 Calorie Plan (page 219), looks like this:

Vitamin A (International units)	12,637
Thiamine (milligrams)	2.0
Riboflavin (milligrams)	2.7
Niacin (milligrams)	27
Vitamin C (milligrams)	186
Vitamin B$_6$ (milligrams)	3.1
Folacin (micrograms)	440

You can see that, on average, this plan provides more than enough vitamins without supplementation. This is generally true for all the plans in this book, with the exception of three vitamins (thiamine, B$_6$, folacin) provided by the 1200 Calorie Plan. The point is that it is very difficult to provide optimal vitamin levels on low-calorie diets (the vitamin content may be much less on the many diets that provide 800 calories per day, for instance). It is for this reason that the overall philosophy of *The California Diet and Exercise Program* aims at gradually increasing food intake, not leaving you for long periods on low-calorie diets. If you stay on the 1200 Calorie Plan for longer than a month (for instance, for Entry Level 1400 calories, page 195), then a daily vitamin-mineral capsule is advisable (one that supplies the RDA but not more). But remember the main point: We want you gradually to play more, so that you can lose weight and gradually eat more and thus not need vitamin supplements — your diet will supply the vitamins you need.

MINERALS

Minerals are essential elements needed in the diet. They are needed for many functions, including some well-known "construction" jobs: adequate calcium (for healthy bones), adequate iron (for healthy blood).

The major minerals considered in constructing our diets are as follows (with the adult male RDA in familiar units):

Calcium	(800 milligrams)
Phosphorus	(800 milligrams)
Magnesium	(350 milligrams)

Iron	(10 milligrams for men;
	18 milligrams for women)
Zinc	(15 milligrams)

The adult male RDA generally equals or exceeds the adult female RDA, with one exception: The female RDA for iron is set at 18 milligrams per day. This relates to the need to replace iron lost in menstruation in women.

The mineral section of the Nutritional Content for the 2400 Calorie Plan (page 223) looks like this:

Calcium (milligrams)	1206
Phosphorus (milligrams)	1781
Magnesium (milligrams)	558
Iron (milligrams)	22
Zinc (milligrams)	18

For this plan, all mineral contents exceed the RDAs, and this is generally true except for zinc and iron in the 1200 Calorie Plan (page 206), which are borderline. Again, a vitamin-mineral capsule supplement is recommended for anyone remaining on the 1200 Calorie Plan for more than one month.

It should be noted that it is unrealistic to be *too* slavish about RDAs. The values assigned to RDAs are intentionally liberal; and our limited ability to measure portion sizes, plus the variability of vitamin and mineral content from batch to batch of a food product, all contribute to the approximate nature of the extremely useful RDA system. To be on the safe side, increase your play and work up to the higher calorie intakes! You can get the vitamins and minerals you need by eating a variety of foods from all the food groups.

Silly Supplements

Supplementation of our food supply with capsules and pills is a major industry. Estimates of the proportion of Americans who regularly take vitamin, mineral and other supplements range from 40 to 70 percent. There are, of course, some circumstances in which supplementation is desirable or even vital; these circumstances should be indicated by a qualified dietitian or physician. The vast majority of other "do-it-yourself" supplementation, supported by massive advertising, has little, if any, scientific underpinning, and in some circumstances can be dangerous. The water-soluble vitamins, for instance, cannot be stored in the body, and so must be excreted in the urine as fast as they can be swallowed. The fat-soluble vitamins, on the other hand, can be stored in the liver and elsewhere, and so may accumulate to dangerously high levels if long-term supplementation at high levels occurs. Further research is needed to determine what harmful consequences such large doses of the vitamins may have on metabolic processes. For example, large amounts of vitamin C can interfere with vitamin B_{12} absorption and metabolism in man. The aim of virtually all nutritional experts today is to persuade the vast majority of Americans to eat enough of a nutritious diet so that supplementation is not necessary. Increasing play level, as we have seen, is a vital part of this process. In view of this, the reports of some fitness exponents taking literally hundreds of supplements each day represent a rather profound difference between theory and practice.

For many people, the daily vitamin-mineral supplement is merely a modestly expensive way of "covering all bases," of trying to be sure there are no deficiences. But, of course, this is tantamount to admitting that your usual diet is inadequate, and leaves something to be desired. It is certainly possible that daily consumption of very large amounts (megadoses) of some vitamin or mineral may, one day, be shown to be of considerable health benefit. And there are some indications of benefit in some instances, that are now attracting the attention of researchers. But there remains a huge national consumption of silly supplements, from bee pollen to kelp, that have no scientific basis.

Vegetarianism

It seems unlikely that man was intended to be a vegetarian, although some of his evolutionary cousins are. The all-vegetable diet certainly has a number of important health attributes, especially relating to heart disease and cancer; and a move toward vegetarianism would almost certainly benefit the American population from the health standpoint. On the other hand, it becomes increasingly important to watch carefully for nutritional content as a diet becomes more and more strictly vegetarian. This applies particularly to protein quality and to adequate amounts of calcium, iron, riboflavin and vitamin B_{12}. This book is not designed for strict vegetarians, and so these particular concerns do not arise with our diets. For readers who are vegetarian, or are considering becoming so, the Reference section contains some articles covering nutritional adequacy on these diets.

Vitamins, Minerals and Cancer

The food supply might contribute to the overall cancer problem in a population in two ways: by adding some substance or substances that cause or promote cancers, and by adding some substance or substances that prevent or hinder development of cancers. Clear but rare examples of the first case are demonstrated in animals, where a particular dietary component causes a specific cancer (for instance, aflatoxin produced by the fungus on stored peanuts has caused liver cancer in ducks and turkeys). Suspicions exist for human populations: nitrites in food are of concern, since they can be converted to carcinogenic nitrosamines; and we have already looked at the *association* between the habitual consumption of fat and meat in world populations, and the incidence of breast and colon cancers.

The possibility that the presence of specific entities in the diet may *prevent* certain cancers ("Chemoprevention") is cause for much scientific excitement and activity at this time. There is by no means general agreement about the potential for dietary manipulation of cancer risk. A report issued in 1980 entitled *Toward Healthful Diets* (Food and Nutrition Board of the National Academy of Sciences) found that no causal relationship had been proved between nutrition and any type of cancer, and so there was no basis to recommend any modification of diet. However, a report issued by the National Research Council in July 1982, entitled *Diet, Nutrition and Cancer,* states, "It is highly likely that the United States will eventually have the option of adopting a diet that reduces its incidence of cancer by approximately one-third." Modest dietary changes were recommended.

These apparently divergent statements reflect different panel reactions to the *same* data, although some new reports were available to the later panel. Neither report recommends supplementation of the diet with pills, but the later report emphasizes daily inclusion of fruits, vegetables and whole grain cereal products in the diet. This recommendation is based on a considerable number of studies showing that people consuming low levels of vitamin A and/or the orange pigment carotene (which is converted into vitamin A in the intestine) were somewhat more likely to develop cancer at various sites (lung, stomach, bladder, prostate) than people consuming higher levels. The differences were not of great magnitude, ranging up to three times the risk for the low-intake groups. This is a much less "powerful" effect than that attributable to smoking (rather than not smoking), in the case of lung cancer. In laboratory experiments with animals, there is evidence that beta carotene, vitamin C, the mineral selenium and various chemicals present in cabbage, Brussels sprouts and broccoli, may protect against the development of cancer.

The degree of interest in chemoprevention (especially for high-risk individuals such as smokers) is such that a large-scale four-year trial is in progress in the United States, involving many thousands of male physicians aged 40 to 75. The participants will take either a beta carotene capsule or a placebo (a look-alike capsule containing an inert substance) each day. It is hoped that this trial will prove (or disprove) the value of beta carotene supplementation in reducing cancer risk.

How does all this relate to *The California Diet*? The following nutritionally excellent foods, among many others, contain several of the vitamins, minerals or other components that *may* reduce cancer risk if eaten regularly:

Apricots
Broccoli
Brussels sprouts
Cantaloupes
Carrots
Peaches
Tomatoes

Did you know that California is the No. 1 U.S. producer of each of these items? Their regular consumption has been recommended by a blue-ribbon committee of the National Research Council, and you will find them cropping up all the time in our menu plans and recipes. Levels of vitamin A, which include beta carotene's contribution, and vitamin C are noted in the nutritional content for each calorie plan.

FIBER

Dietary fiber is the name given to a group of substances in our diet that contribute to the structure of vegetable foods, and are indigestible. They provide very little energy, and so tended to be ignored until recent years as a "useless" part of our diet. Dietary fiber is a mixture of different types of compound. Some dissolve in water (pectins and gums), but others do not (cellulose, hemicellulose, lignins). Some of the major sources of natural dietary fiber are:

• Whole grains.
• Fresh fruits, especially apples, pears and berries.
• Fresh vegetables, especially artichokes, broccoli, carrots, corn, potatoes and squash.
• Dried fruits, nuts and seeds.
• Cooked dried beans (kidney, navy and garbanzo).

The health-promoting virtues of dietary fiber have been extolled in recent years, notably by Dr. Dennis Burkitt of London. A recent study, reported in September 1982, related to fiber intake among 871 middle-aged men in the town of Zutphen, Netherlands. Information on their food intake was collected, and they were then followed (the time course method) for 10 years. Death rate from heart attacks was four times higher in the men on the lowest intake of dietary fiber, when compared to men on the highest intake, but the cancer death rate was three times higher for the men on the lowest intake. It is noteworthy that some good sources of fiber (fruits, dark green and orange vegetables) are also good sources of beta carotene, so that an association with higher intakes of beta carotene might be the actual cause of the "protective" effect of fiber seen in this study.

There is at least some persuasive evidence, for at least some forms of dietary fiber, of the following health benefits associated with a high-fiber diet:

- Reduced or eliminated constipation
- Prevention of hemorrhoids
- Prevention or improvement of diverticular disease
- Better control of diabetes
- Reduction of plasma total cholesterol levels.

The evidence for more spectacular claims made for high-fiber diets — prevention of colon cancer, heart disease and appendicitis — is quite indirect and at present not very persuasive.

In considering the well-constructed diet, we have aimed at menu plans providing generous (13 grams or more) dietary fiber contents through the liberal use of natural sources (fruits, vegetables, grains). The current consensus is that fiber should be obtained from the basic foods for a diet, rather than sprinkled on as a powder, or eaten as a pill.

In the light of what we currently know about vitamins, minerals and fiber, a well-constructed diet should contain adequate amounts of the essential vitamins and minerals, generous amounts of some of the vitamins that may relate to risk of developing cancer, and a generous supply of fiber. All of these things should come packaged in regular, appetizing foods, rather than as supplements. This is what you will find in the menu plans and recipes of *The California Diet*. We want you to lose weight sensibly and permanently, but we are also concerned about your future health and good food habits.

11. Dietary Villains?

The dietitian has one further task: to consider the place of several common dietary components that have been at the center of some king-sized arguments in recent years. These controversial characters are:

- Alcohol
- Caffeine
- Cholesterol
- Salt
- Sugar

They are a mixed bunch. One is essential (salt); two provide energy (alcohol and sugar); three are perfectly natural, and have been part of the diet of millions for centuries (cholesterol, salt and sugar); and two are drugs (caffeine and alcohol).

Whenever there is uncertainty, there will be many strongly held opinions — perhaps in a worthy cause — since, according to the English poet Milton, "opinion in good men is but knowledge in the making."

Let's look briefly, then, at the various facets of this controversial nutritional quintet.

ALCOHOL

History. Undoubtedly, alcohol in one form or another has been a significant dietary component for most populations since time immemorial. It differs from other dietary components in several important respects: Some members of a population will consume large amounts, whereas others will consume none at all; there are strong moral and religious feelings and proscriptions about the use of alcohol; it is intoxicating, and it contributes a sizeable proportion of total calories to the diet of many people, without benefit of accompanying nutrients.

167

Drinking alcohol is a widespread habit, of course. In 1982, 65 percent of adult Americans said they drank alcoholic beverages; true use may be higher. Drinking rates are not homogenous across the country: In California the adult drinking rate (1982) was 77 percent. Recently there has been a small decline in proportion of drinkers nationwide (from a high of 71 percent in 1978), according to statistics.

Attempts to prohibit, or decrease, drinking have historically been remarkably unsuccessful, at least within democratic societies. Looked at realistically, alcohol consumption must be seen as a significant part of dietary intake for many people, and it seems likely to remain that way for years to come.

The Good. Even scientists look over their shoulders before saying good things about alcohol, such is the strength of feeling about its immoderate use. Nonetheless, we must take a balanced view of all dietary components. Alcohol is a central nervous system depressant (not a stimulant). The relaxation and enhanced sociability produced rapidly by alcohol endear it to millions; its dispensation is a virtually routine part of business, professional and social gatherings. Recent studies have shown that individuals who drink regularly, but not heavily (one to three drinks, or up to about two ounces of pure alcohol per day), suffer fewer deaths from coronary heart disease than non-drinkers. Since coronary heart disease is still our major cause of death, we have to say that the evidence is that "moderate" drinking reduces death rate from our No. 1 killer. In recent studies by Dr. Joseph Barboriak and Dr. Harvey Gruchow and their colleagues, during which the condition of the coronary arteries was examined by X-ray techniques (coronary arteriography) in large numbers of men, it was found that regular drinkers had "cleaner" coronary arteries than either occasional drinkers or non-drinkers. Cigarette smoking was predictably associated with increased coronary artery disease, so that the non-smoking alcohol abstainers showed about the same amount of artery disease as heavy smokers consuming more than six ounces of alcohol per week. The men with the greatest amount of disease were the non-drinking heavy smokers, those with the least amount, the non-smoking drinkers.

The mechanism of the apparently "protective" effect of regular alcohol intake with respect to coronary heart disease is not clear. Alcohol increases the concentration of HDL (high-density lipoprotein) particles in the blood (see page 132), and this may represent another association of higher levels of HDL with lower heart disease rates. However, the biochemistry involved here is not simple, and further studies are needed to clarify the situation.

The Bad. Now the bad news. Alcohol is a drug. It may well be that it is a relatively effective drug for the specific purpose of reducing coronary heart disease in the United States. Unlike most drugs, in their social obscurity, alcohol is not sold on prescription, in small bottles at the pharmacy; rather, it is sold without prescription, in large bottles at the liquor store. But like virtually all drugs, it has side effects.

The list of negative effects of alcohol is long and "sobering." Immoderate use is strongly associated with vehicular deaths and homicide, with family problems and addiction, with cirrhosis of the liver (a leading cause of death) and with increased blood pressure and more frequent problems of heart rhythm. Alcohol use during pregnancy increases risk of damage to the fetus. Actually, the list is about as long and depressing as the catalog of side effects found, written in small print, on the package insert for many modern drugs. In other words, alcohol is a drug with high public acceptance that can have severe side effects, including addiction, especially when taken in high doses for many, many years.

Although alcohol use is associated with lessened coronary heart disease, it is also associated with increased incidence of various cancers, especially when combined with smoking. Increased rates of cancer of the mouth, pharynx, larynx and esophagus are found in smoking drinkers. Pure alcohol is not carcinogenic; but it may be that the solvent action of alcohol (especially in the form of the stronger spirits) enables carcinogenic materials in cigarette smoke to gain closer access to cells of these target organs.

The reasonable conclusion from these considerations is well stated in *Dietary Guidelines for Americans:* "If you drink alcohol, do so in moderation." In *The California Diet* we do not advocate drinking alcohol. It is clear that the moderate drinker frequently avoids all of the "side effects" mentioned above. Remember that alcohol provides calories without nutrients. The calorie plans in this book do not feature alcoholic drinks, but you can include them if you wish by using Exchange List J (pages 248-250).

CAFFEINE

History. Caffeine is one of a family of compounds called xanthines. The main U.S. sources are coffee, the cola drinks, tea, chocolate, cocoa and certain over-the-counter drugs. Caffeine is a central nervous system stimulant — the opposite of alcohol. Taking caffeine, for instance in coffee, rapidly increases pulse rate, blood pressure, and the amount of free fatty acids circulating in the blood. The degree of stimulation tends to wear off in regular users, so that the greatest effect is in people not used to regular doses of caffeine. Americans consume large quantities of caffeine, although there is a movement toward decaffeinated coffees and virtually caffeine-free colas. But an estimated 20 to 30 percent of Americans consume 500 to 600 milligrams of caffeine daily (one cup of coffee contains about 120 milligrams caffeine). Over half of the world's coffee is sold to the United States; and the average consumption of cola beverages is now an astonishing 30 gallons per capita per year.

The Good. The caffeine-containing drinks certainly have their social values, although these can be preserved in the absence of caffeine. The stimulant action of coffee and colas is valuable in some circumstances.

The Bad. Consumption of moderate doses of caffeine does not have profound, acute, adverse health effects. But for some people, in some circumstances, caffeine use may promote sleeplessness, rapid or irregular heart beat, frequent urination and jitteriness, among other effects.

In the long term, regular consumption of caffeine may have more serious health effects, but the evidence is certainly not strong. Blood pressure may be somewhat higher overall as a result of taking caffeine regularly, although the effect appears to "wear off" with regular use. Regular coffee use has been thought to be associated with increased risk of death from coronary disease, but currently there is very little good evidence for this. Coffee drinking has also been associated with increased risk of cancer of the pancreas, whereas tea drinking did not show the association (although tea contains caffeine). But the evidence available on the coffee-pancreatic cancer issue is still inadequate to cause serious concern. The question deserves further study.

On balance, there is more to be said for avoiding caffeine than for regularly consuming it, although the evidence against moderate caffeine consumption as a health hazard is relatively weak in comparison to some dietary components. Scientific and government reports of recent years, in making recommendations for dietary change in America, have generally ignored the question of caffeine consumption.

Frequent consumption of coffee, tea and cola drinks is not recommended or included in *The California Diet.* Some studies have shown an association between caffeine consumption during pregnancy and birth defects. Fibrocystic breast disease in women has also been linked to caffeine consumption. These associations deserve further study. These items often provide calories (particularly sugar) without accompanying nutrients. If you incorporate coffee, tea or cola drinks into your diet, remember the calories that often go with them!

CHOLESTEROL

History. Cholesterol, a moderately complex, widely occurring steroidal alcohol, has promoted thousands of news stories, a great deal of sponsored scientific research and numerous bad jokes. Spelling and prononunication of the word have improved immensely in recent years.

Cholesterol was known by scientists to be circulating in our blood before the California gold rush of 1849, so it's not a new topic. Biologically, cholesterol exists only in animals, so a strict vegetarian diet is "cholesterol free." Cholesterol is vital to animal life: It forms part of cell membranes and is very prominent in the brain and nerves; it is also the raw material for production of cortisol, the sex hormones and the bile acids (which help digest fat). Most tissues of the body can *make* their own cholesterol, so that in non-vegetarians the five ounces or so of cholesterol in the average human body have come partly from the diet, partly from the body's own manufacture.

Cholesterol is in a constant state of flux. New molecules are added through dietary intake and body synthesis, and this is balanced by loss of cholesterol, and the bile acids made from it, in the stool. Dietary cholesterol *tends* to increase the level of cholesterol in the bloodstream (both the LDL and the HDL particles — see page 132), although the amount of cholesterol in the diet is by no means the only determinant of blood cholesterol level. Diets rich in saturated fat tend to *increase* LDL levels, as diets rich in polyunsaturated (usually liquid vegetable) fats tend to *decrease* LDL.

The finding by Anitschkow (1913), in Russia, that cholesterol fed to rabbits produced lesions in their arteries that resembled human coronary artery disease, sparked an enormous interest in all aspects of the structure, metabolism and epidemiology of cholesterol, which continues to this day.

The Good. In spite of its usually bad press, cholesterol is a vital, versatile substance that we *must* have. We just don't want too much in the wrong place. We do not *require* cholesterol in the diet, since it is not a vitamin for humans. The vegetarian gorilla, for instance, is robust and has plenty of cholesterol in his body — he has made it all himself. But *modest* amounts of cholesterol in the diet are quite compatible with good health and freedom from coronary disease.

The Bad. Too much cholesterol in the bloodstream, in the form of LDL particles, is clearly a strong risk factor for coronary disease. Individuals with extremely high LDL levels, resulting from a genetic defect, typically (if not successfully treated) succumb to heart attacks by age 20. There is an enormous amount of epidemiological evidence pointing to unnaturally high blood levels of LDL-cholesterol as a leading cause of coronary heart disease. There has been some interest recently in the possibility that *low* levels of blood cholesterol may be associated with *increased* levels of cancer. It's only a theory, but considerable research is going on in this area.

Since it is advisable, with our present knowledge, to keep our blood LDL at reasonably low levels, the important question here is: How much influence is dietary cholesterol going to have on our LDL levels? Although it is true that our bodies have some capacity to turn down their production rate of cholesterol to balance dietary intake, a reasonably low dietary cholesterol intake is advisable to maintain low LDL levels. This has been a rather unfortunate conclusion to reach, since many dietary items (e.g., eggs and liver) are rich in cholesterol, but are also excellent sources of important nutrients.

Dietary Guidelines for Americans, Recommendation No. 3, reads: "Avoid too much fat, saturated fat, and cholesterol." The plea for *moderation* sums up the scientific consensus about this controversial subject. You will find this recommendation reflected in the menu plans in this book. We have tried to keep average daily cholesterol intake below 300 milligrams per day (see Nutritional Contents for each plan) by using high-cholesterol animal foods in moderation, and emphasizing use of cholesterol-free oils and fruits and vegetables, breads and legumes.

SALT

History. Some salt in the diet is essential to our health. In fact, the salt trade has been extremely important, historically, because of the need for salt by peoples in inland areas where salt is not locally available. Salt is the major source of sodium, a mineral. An extremely important aspect of salt in our past history has been its use as a preservative for fish, meat and other products. Salting made perishable foods available for consumption through the winter. Probably because of this widespread use of salt for preserving and curing foods, we have come to accept — even expect — an unnaturally salty taste in association with many products. This is an acquired taste (not shared by most animals; my dog rejects salted peanuts but loves salt-free nuts) that can be altered fairly rapidly. Many processed foods contain extremely high quantities of salt (most soups, canned meats, for instance). It is easy to withdraw salt gradually from the diet so that return to a can of salted soup is an unpleasant experience. A considerable number of unsalted or low-salt items are beginning to appear in food stores, as America gradually realizes that we have freezers to preserve food, and can now kick the "salt habit." Baby foods are lower in salt than was once the case.

The Good. Salt certainly does enhance the flavor of some foods for many people, but other flavorings can be more subtle and, often, simply better. More importantly, sodium is an essential mineral. But many Americans eat 10 to 20 times the amount of sodium they actually need, so substantial reductions can safely be recommended for most people.

The Bad. Why worry about salt if you like it? There is gradually increasing evidence that high blood pressure is worsened (and may even be caused) by chronic high salt intake. Populations with naturally low-salt intakes show very little hypertension. Many studies have shown improvements in the blood pressures of hypertensive people simply by reduction of salt intake, especially in those whose genetic makeup predisposes them to hypertension. Now, of course, we can treat hypertension with a variety of drugs (all with some side effects). But it seems prudent to help nature as much as we can by reducing salt intake, and then considering drug treatment if this is still necessary. There is a reasonable possibility that a low salt intake, begun early in life, may protect persons at risk of developing hypertension.

Various gastrointestinal cancers have been associated with heavy intake of foods that have been salt-cured or smoked.

Recommendation No. 6 of *Dietary Guidelines for Americans* states: Avoid too much sodium.

- Learn to enjoy the unsalted flavors of foods.
- Cook with only small amounts of added salt.
- Add little or no salt to food at the table.
- Limit your intake of salty foods, such as potato chips, pretzels, salted nuts and popcorn, condiments (soy sauce, steak sauce, garlic salt), cheese, pickled foods, cured meats.
- Read food labels carefully to determine the amounts of sodium in processed foods and snack items.

The diets in this book are constructed to be moderately low in salt. The Nutritional Contents do not show salt content, because this can be influenced greatly by salt added at the table. We recommend not adding salt from the shaker or during cooking, unless this is specifically mentioned in the recipes. Very similar food products can vary enormously in salt content, so read labels when buying processed cereals and canned meats, soups and vegetables.

SUGAR

History. Sugar (or sucrose) is a naturally occurring, simple carbohydrate. In the early 1900s, sugar contributed 12 percent to total U.S. calories, but this has increased to 18 percent today. The increase is largely due to the addition of refined sugar (from sugar beet and sugar cane) to manufactured foods and beverages — pies, ice cream, sweetened soft drinks, etc. About 100 pounds of sugar per capita is consumed annually in America, or about one quarter pound each day for every person in the country. We spend more than $5 billion a year on soft drinks in the United States, which buys us water, sugar, flavoring and sometimes coloring and caffeine. As with salt, our taste preference has been "trained" by the products generally available and provided to us in cafeterias, restaurants, airplanes and our own homes.

The Good. People like sweet foods. Sugar is a cheap, rapid source of energy.

The Bad. The major, clear health problem with high-sugar intake is promotion of tooth decay, especially in children. In spite of considerable discussion over the years, the consensus is that a high-sugar diet is not directly responsible for the onset of either diabetes or heart disease. A possible health hazard relates to the "empty" nature of calories provided by refined sugar. Empty calories are calories that do not provide us with vitamins, minerals or protein. A diet high in refined sugar will tend to displace other nutritious food items, in particular the complex carbohydrates, vitamins, minerals and fiber that are contained in fruits and vegetables.

Recommendation No. 5 of *Dietary Guidelines for Americans* states: "Avoid too much sugar."

To avoid excessive sugars:

• Use less of all sugars, including white sugar, brown sugar, raw sugar, honey and syrups.

• Eat less of foods containing these sugars, such as candy, soft drinks, ice cream, cakes, cookies.

• Select fresh fruits or fruits canned without sugar or with light syrup, rather than heavy syrup.

• Read food labels for clues on sugar content; if the name sucrose, glucose, maltose, dextrose, lactose, fructose or syrup appears first, then there is a large amount of sugar.

• Remember, how often you eat sugar is as important as how much sugar you eat.

The plans in *The California Diet* have been constructed to be low in refined sugar. The Nutritional Contents indicate that this component is held at about 10 grams or less per day. Remember that addition of items from Exchange List J may add considerable amounts of refined sugar. Where possible, read the label!

12. The California Foods

California is a wonderland of exciting foods — the major U.S. producer of many interesting and healthy offerings from almonds to walnuts, from apricots to tomatoes. Of course, we have featured many of these foods, especially the fruits and vegetables, in the healthful menu plans of *The California Diet*.

In this chapter you will find out more about these foods:

• California's leading fruits and vegetables; harvest season and economic importance.

• Efficient selection, storage and preparation of California produce.

• California commodities; some things you might like to know about 16 important fruits and vegetables.

Bon Appetit!

CALIFORNIA COMMODITIES

California agriculture is considered one of the most diversified in the world, with no one crop dominating the state's farm economy. Most crops individually account for less than 2 percent of the state's total gross farm income. California leads the nation by a wide margin in the production of fruits, nuts and vegetables; it accounts for more than 40 percent of the nation's cash farm receipts for fruits and nuts, and about one-third for vegetables.

Some 200 crops are recognized in California, including seeds, flowers and ornamentals. Sixty-nine major crops are grown on a commercial scale in California with 45 of these accounting for most of the U.S. production. This section includes information on 16 produce items for your reference. These specific foods were chosen for discussion for one or more of the following reasons:

• Outstanding nutritional quality (especially those foods that contain nutrients shown to be marginal in many diets, i.e., vitamins A and C, and the mineral iron).

• Current topic of research in health.

• Good economy and availability.

• Special knowledge needed in purchasing for quality.

• Special storage instructions.

Much of the following information on California commodities was obtained from *The Packer's Produce Availability and Merchandising Guide, 1982,* and from the various California produce advisory boards.

Almonds

Care: Most nuts will store for up to 12 months under proper storage conditions. Prevent nuts from picking up moisture, and do not store nuts with any commodity that has a strong odor, such as fresh fruits, onions, potatoes or meat. Packaged nuts will hold up well at room temperatures, but should be stored in cool, dry places if they are to be held for any length of time.

Nutrition: Virtually all nutrition education programs now emphasize consuming more vegetable protein sources and fewer animal protein sources in our diets. The reason for this is that animal foods tend to be high in saturated fat and cholesterol, and foods from plants contain mainly unsaturated fat and no cholesterol and tend to be sources of nutrients that are sometimes deficient in American diets. However, you must beware of consuming too many nuts, if on a low-calorie diet. Almonds (54 percent fat by weight) have a lot of energy: 170 calories per ounce.

The nutrient composition of almonds is as follows.

• *Fat:* Seventy-nine percent of the calories are from fat. However, this fat is highly unsaturated, having a polyunsaturated to saturated fat (P/S) ratio of 3.0.

• *Protein:* Plant-source protein, such as almonds, is desirable because it is accompanied by little saturated fat and contains no cholesterol. One ounce of almonds supplies about 10 percent of the Recommended Daily Allowance (RDA). However, this is not a complete protein and must be combined with either grains, legumes, or milk products to equal the protein quality of meat. Comparatively, a one-ounce serving of meat supplies about 13 percent of the RDA for protein.

- *Carbohydrate:* Almond carbohydrate, like potato and other vegetable carbohydrate, is largely of the "complex" type (as distinguished from simple sugars in fruits).

- *Fiber:* Although no requirement has been established for fiber, nutritionists recommend that most Americans increase their daily intake. One ounce of almonds will supply approximately 0.6 grams of fiber, about equal to two slices of whole wheat bread.

- *Vitamins:* Almonds contain a significant amount of several vitamins. They are an excellent source of vitamin E; a one-ounce serving supplies 35 percent of the U.S. RDA. Riboflavin is also present in good amounts; a one-ounce serving supplies approximately 15 percent of the RDA. Almonds also contain smaller amounts of thiamine, niacin and folacin.

- *Minerals:* Almonds contain trace amounts of copper and magnesium. A one-ounce serving of almonds also supplies approximately 8 percent of the RDA for calcium and iron.

Uses: Almonds are used quite often in our recipes and menu plans. They are used in fruit salads, hot and cold cereals, vegetable and meat salads, hot vegetables (almondine), stir-fried, and baked entrees, pastas, rice, and many desserts. Almonds also make a great snack, served with fresh or dried fruit.

Requests for recipes can be directed to: Almond Board of California, P.O. Box 15920, Sacramento, CA 95852. Include a self-addressed, stamped envelope.

Apricots

The apricot began about 4000 years ago in China, where the fruit still grows wild in the mountains, and followed the wanderings of man to all parts of the globe. With the Spaniards, the apricot traveled to the New World in the 15th and 16th centuries. Seedlings were planted at the Spanish missions in California in the 18th century. Commercial cultivation of apricots in California started in 1792 from an orchard in the town of Santa Clara. Today, California is one of the major apricot-producing areas in the world, and accounts for 97 percent of U.S. apricots. Approach of harvest is signalled by the annual apricot fiesta in the bountiful San Joaquin Valley.

Nutrition: Apricots are low in calories, but high in nutritional value (thereby making them a nutrient-dense food). Two fresh apricots provide 38 percent of the adult recommended dietary allowance of vitamin A, 12 percent of vitamin C, and only 36 calories. Apricots are also a significant source of potassium. Six pounds of fresh apricots are needed to make one pound of dried fruit, so that dried apricots are concentrated in flavor and nutrition. Dried apricots are an especially good source of iron, providing two milligrams per 100 calories. The nutritional superiority of apricots was recognized by NASA officials who included dried apricots in the menu for the astronauts on the Gemini and Mercury space flights.

Uses: For weight-reducing diets, add apricots to recipes for a natural, sweet flavor in place of syrup, sugar or honey. When pureed or mashed, apricots become thick and creamy, a good substitute for fats and creams in many recipes. Apricots are particularly well-suited for desserts and salads, as well as meat dishes, glazes, and beverages.

Many recipes have evolved from the apricot harvest festival recipe competition, as well as from the kitchens of apricot grower families. For a booklet containing these recipes, as well as recipes for special diets, including diabetic, low-cholesterol, high-fiber, and low-sodium, write to: California Apricot Advisory Board, 1280 Boulevard Way, Walnut Creek, CA 94595. Information may also be obtained on drying, freezing and canning apricots.

Avocados

Care: Avocados are not as tempermental as some other fruits. Avocados never soften on the tree, although they must be allowed to reach full maturity before being picked, in order to develop their full flavor. The tree acts as a storehouse, so the avocado can be held on the tree for months, developing fully in flavor and maturity.

Some folks say money doesn't grow on trees. However, if you are lucky enough to have a few avocado trees in your backyard, like some of my friends, the trees can offer support during tax time, with very little investment.

The best avocados are generally free from bruises. Appearance may be marred, however, by irregular markings known as "scab," which is superficial and does not affect the flavor or flesh. Soft-skinned green varieties that are turning black or that have black spots probably will be soft and mushy and should be avoided. Finger marks indicate bad areas beneath the skin.

To test for ripeness, cradle the fruit in the hand. If it is soft to the touch, it is probably ripe. If it is hard, ripening can be advanced by placing the avocado in a brown paper bag or wrapping in foil, and leaving at room temperature.

To prevent darkening once an avocado has been cut, it may be brushed with lemon or lime juice. Unused, cut avocados should be stored in air-tight wrap with the seed replaced.

Many people grow their own avocado plant from the seed. Just place three toothpicks in a circular fashion around the center of the seed. Prop the seed in a glass of water so that half of the seed is immersed in water at all times and half out of water. With patience, the seed will form roots, and can then be planted in soil. Again, place only half the seed in the soil and leave the other half exposed to the air. In time a nice indoor plant will emerge.

Nutrition: Unlike most fruits that are high in carbohydrates, avocados can contain as much as 17 percent oil (by total weight of edible fruit). The Fuerte avocado is higher in fat than the Haas, as you can probably tell by its creamier texture. The fat content of avocados provides 76 to 89 percent of their total calories, which is why they are listed in the fat exchange list. But, avocados are rich in unsaturated oil and contain no cholesterol, which makes them a good food on the fat exchange list for low-cholesterol or low-saturated fat diets. Avocados also have trace amounts of vitamins A and E, thiamine and riboflavin.

Broccoli

Care: The best broccoli will have a firm, compact cluster of small flower buds. None should be open enough to reveal the yellow flowers inside. The clusters should be dark or sage green and may have a purplish cast to them. Broccoli that is yellowish-green in color or wilted in appearance generally will be overmature and should be avoided.

Nutrition: Nutritionally, broccoli is a very good buy. One-half cup of cooked broccoli stalks, cut into one-half-inch pieces, provides 34 percent of the RDA of vitamin A for an adult. The same amount will provide the daily allowance of vitamin C and significant amounts of iron. All that nutrition is yours for only 26 calories!

Uses: After trimming away any woody portions of the stem, quarter the stalk, so that it will cook in the same time as the flower buds. Steaming broccoli is the best way to preserve its nutritional value. Also, leave the lid slightly ajar to allow the steam to escape in order to preserve the nice green color of the broccoli. This allows the volatile acids to escape, which otherwise turn the broccoli to an army gray-green color. (Note, however, that *overcooked* broccoli will still turn color). Broccoli can then be topped with any dressing, or lemon juice, margarine, nuts, herbs or spices.

Carrots

Care: Most carrots today are sold without tops. Tops have been shown to withdraw moisture from the roots, so carrots without tops will store better. A good carrot should be firm, smooth and well-colored. Carrots with large green areas at the top are undesirable. Badly shaped carrots can cause excessive waste during the preparation process.

Nutrition: Carrots are an excellent source of vitamin A. One-half cup of carrots (about 100 grams) can supply twice the average adult RDA of vitamin A. The darker the orange color of the carrot, the more vitamin A it contains. Carrots retain their vitamin A content well in storage.

The orange pigment of carrots is called carotene, which is converted to vitamin A in the body. Carotene is of considerable interest today since it may play a role in preventing certain types of cancer (see Chapter 10).

Dates

California and Arizona are the chief date growing states, although some come from Texas, Florida and the Gulf states. Dates are also imported from Iraq.

Care: Deglet Noor and similar varieties (semi-dry) require a temperature of 32°F to best retain flavor, texture, color and aroma. They will hold for one year at 32° and somewhat longer at 0°. Dates of the soft, invert-sugar type (Khadrawy, Zahidi, Halawy) should be refrigerated at all times. Soft dates will hold for six months at 32° and for one year at 0°.

Generally, dates should be soft with smooth texture. Refrigerate dates in sealed containers to keep them from absorbing odors.

Nutrition: Dates are about 73 percent sugar and have been called "candy that grows on trees." Though different varieties contain different types of sugar (sucrose versus dextrose and glucose), there is essentially no difference in the human metabolism. Along with this naturally sweet delight comes small amounts of iron (one milligram per 100 calories). If dates are used as a natural source of sugar to sweeten breads, cookies, cereals and salads, they will serve a useful purpose in adding nutritional value, too.

For further information on dates contact: California Date Administrative Committee, 81855 Highway 111, Room 2-G, Indio, CA 92201.

Grapes

Preserved grape seeds found with remains of the Bronze Age, and Egyptian murals describing grape growing around 2440 B.C. are testimony to the role played by grapes in the life of early man. When the Vikings landed in North America they christened the new land "Vinland" in honor of the abundance of native grapes. European varieties were brought to the eastern United States by English settlers, but the vines could not withstand the harsh climate. Spanish missionaries introduced grape vines throughout California and by 1860, the commercial grape growing venture in California was underway. Today, California produces more than 91 percent of the nation's supply of table grapes.

Care: Storage characteristics of grapes vary depending on the particular variety and the quality of the grape. European types will store much longer than American types, and both should be refrigerated.

Stem coloring provides a good indication of storage quality. Well-matured stems of light green or straw color generally store well. Grapes are sensitive to damage and should be handled carefully. The white varieties, particularly, are easily damaged. Grapes that are well-colored, plump, and firmly attached to the stem are generally of good quality. White or green grapes will have a yellowish cast or straw color with a touch of amber when they are at their taste peak. Red varieties are best when all of the berries are predominantly red.

Avoid grapes that are soft or wrinkled, as they may have been frozen or overdried. A bleached area around the stem indicates injury and poor quality.

Nutrition: Grapes are a good snack food for those who are dieting. Grapes are naturally sweet, and one cup contains approximately 100 calories and provides approximately 10 percent of the RDA for vitamin C. Grapes supply necessary fiber.

For further information on grapes, along with a consumer recipe book, send a self-addressed, stamped envelope to: California Table Grape Commission, P.O. Box 5498, Fresno, CA 93755, (209) 224-4997.

Legumes

Varieties: Legume is a general term referring to dried beans, peas, and lentils. Although you may not find all of the varieties on the grocery shelf, here are some of the more popular varieties and their uses:

Beans

Black beans (or black turtle soup beans): Used in thick soups and oriental and Mediterranean dishes.

Black-eye peas (also called black-eye beans or cow-peas): These beans are small, oval-shaped, and creamy white with a black spot on one side, used as a main-dish vegetable.

Garbanzo beans (or chick-peas): Light tan-colored with a nut-like flavor; commonly pickled in vinegar and oil for salads. Also used as a main dish vegetable or in Middle Eastern dishes. Similar beans are cranberry and yellow-eye beans.

Great Northern beans: Larger than, but similar to, pea beans; used in soups, salads, casserole dishes, and home-baked beans.

Kidney beans: Large, with a red color and kidney shape. They are popular for chili, salads, and Mexican dishes.

Lima beans: Broad and flat, different sizes. They make an excellent main-dish vegetable, and are used in casseroles.

Navy beans: Navy beans is a broad term that includes Great Northern, pea, flat small white, and small white beans.

Pea beans: Small, oval, and white. Pea beans are favored for home-baked beans, soups and casseroles.

Pinto beans: Pinto beans are of the same species as the kidney and red beans. Beige-colored and speckled, they are used mainly in salads, chili, and Mexican dishes.

Red and Pink Beans: Red and Pink beans are related to the kidney bean. Pink beans have a more delicate flavor than red beans. Both are used in chili and Mexican dishes.

Soybeans: Light tan colored, round-shaped like a large pea. Used in stews, casseroles, and soups. Also made into many products as tofu, tempeh and soymilk.

Peas

Green and yellow whole peas and split peas, although they vary in taste a little, are used interchangeably in many recipes. Dry peas are served plain, with meats and game, in dips, soups, casseroles, croquettes, stuffed peppers, and even souffles.

Lentils

Lentils are light brown and disc-shaped, about the size of a pea. Lentils are excellent with meats, as a sauce for grains, in soups, in gravies and stews, and served chilled as a salad on a lettuce bed.

Care: In purchasing, look for beans, peas, and lentils with a bright color, uniform size, and no visible damage. Sometimes cheaper if purchased in bulk.

Legumes should be stored in tightly covered containers and stored in a dry, cool place (50 to 70°F). They will then keep their quality for several months. Do not mix older with newly purchased legumes; this will result in uneven cooking, since older legumes take longer to cook than fresher ones.

Nutrition: Legumes rank very high on the list of food sources of iron, zinc, magnesium, phosphorus, thiamine, B_6, niacin and folacin. They are fair sources of both calcium and riboflavin.

Legumes are often classified as a meat substitute because of their high protein content (an average serving, about ¾ cup cooked, supplies about 18 percent of the RDA for protein). Although an average serving of legumes furnishes only about half as much protein as an average serving of meat (three ounces), when eaten in combination with grains, nuts or dairy products at the same meal, their protein quality is almost equal to that of meat.[1]

Since legumes are a good source of protein, vitamins and minerals, and are low cost (see discussion below), why don't they contribute more to meeting our daily protein allowance? One common complaint is: "I can't digest beans," because the undigestible carbohydrates in beans lead to intestinal flatulence. Take time to incorporate legumes into your diet. Your intestinal flora will adapt to the new carbohydrate source over time, thus decreasing gas production. Also try different types of legumes; each of us has a different tolerance to each variety. It is important to cook legumes well: Cooking for a long time at a lower heat helps to reduce their flatulence-causing properties. Also, if you use the soaking method of cooking beans, then discard the water before cooking, you will minimize those undesirable digestive symptoms. Be aware, however, that you will also discard some of the vitamins and minerals in this way.

Legumes are another category of food that many people think of as fattening, yet legumes supply an average of 15 calories per gram of protein. (Meat supplies about six to 15 calories per gram of protein). Because of the high fiber content of legumes, they tend to be very filling, which is an added bonus for those on a low-calorie diet.

A third complaint often expressed by individuals in their reluctance to eat legumes is that they do not know how to cook them. The following is a simple guide for cooking beans.

Pressure cooking. Bring the washed beans, and three to four times their volume in water, to a boil in the pressure cooker. Cover and bring to 15 pounds pressure. Cook beans according to timetable below. Cool the pressure cooker immediately under cold running water. Open the cooker and drain the stock from the beans. Soaking or precooking saves a little time, but with pressure cooking it really isn't necessary. A pressure cooker is a real advantage in cooking legumes, since a meal doesn't require as much forethought. Lentils and peas (split and black-eye) tend to foam when cooking, so if

---

[1]For an in-depth discussion of protein complementing, see *Diet For A Small Planet,* by Frances Moore Lappe.

using a pressure cooker, do so with caution. Sometimes adding a little oil to the mixture keeps the foam down. Pressure cooking yields a more tender bean.

Regular cooking. Wash the legumes in cold water, removing any visible stones or other debris. Soak overnight (in the refrigerator) in three times the volume of water; or bring the beans and water to a boil, cover tightly, and let sit for two hours. After soaking, simmer the legumes, partially covered, adding water when necessary according to the following timetable.

TIMETABLE FOR COOKING BEANS

	Regular Cooking (soaked beans)	Pressure Cooking (unsoaked beans)
Black beans, kidney, black-eyed peas, pinto and soy beans	2 hours	20-25 minutes
Mung beans, small red beans	3 hours	30-35 minutes
Garbanzos	4 hours	40-45 minutes
Lentils, split peas	1 hour	10-15 minutes

Note: Always remember to allow for expansion of legumes when cooking. Depending on the kind, one cup of dried yields two to 2¾ cups cooked.

Canned beans and peas are convenient if time is of importance for you in meal preparation. Other differences, however, include an increased cost (two times)[1] and sodium (100 times)[2] in canned beans and peas compared to those freshly prepared from dried.

If, after following the above suggestions, you still find it difficult to incorporate legumes into your diet, you may make substitutions in the meal plans. When this vegetable protein source is eliminated, an additional serving (two ounces) of animal protein should be included without a substantial reduction in nutrients or a significant change in calories (see footnote in Exchange List G). The effect of this substitution on cost is worth noting. One serving of vegetable protein costs about 10 to 22 cents per day, for freshly cooked and canned, respectively. Substituting a serving of meat will increase the

[1]Fresh-cooked beans = 10 cents per ¾ cup serving. Canned beans = 22 cents.

[2]Fresh beans = 3 mg sodium per ¾ cup serving. Canned beans = 300 mg.

cost to 50 cents per serving.[1] Since the diets in this book are form-
ulated to meet the RDA for protein, vitamins, and minerals,
(including a serving of vegetable protein), there is no nutritional
benefit per cost by adding more protein to the diet in the form of
meat.

Melons

The melon is a plant of the cucumber family, which may otherwise be known as a gourd. The varieties of sweet melons include:
cantaloupe, honeydew, casaba, crenshaw, Persian, Santa Claus (or
Christmas), and canary.

Cantaloupes begin to appear in May, have a peak season in July,
and continue into early fall. Honeydew, casaba, crenshaws and Persian melons begin their season in June and peak during the July-
August-September months. The Santa Claus melon is available during the month of December, and a new melon variety, the canary, is
available July through November. All melons may be available into
November in some areas.

Cantaloupe. Cantaloupe is identified by a well-raised, coarse, net
surface on a beige-grayish background. If picked at the right
maturity, cantaloupe will have a smoothly rounded depressed
scar at the stem end. If the cantaloupe is held for two to three
days, the color of the rind will become more yellow, the salmon-
orange colored flesh will soften, and there will be a change in the
flavor and aromatic components.

Honeydew. The shape is bluntly oval and it has a smooth rind.
As it matures, the rind changes from a slick whitish-green to a
creamy-white and feels slightly tacky to the touch. The flesh is
delicate green, juicy, very sweet, and has a fine-grained texture. It
has a delicate, sweet, pleasant aroma. The fruit averages $3\frac{1}{3}$ to
seven pounds.

Casaba. The casaba is a winter variety melon with globular shape
and pointed at the stem end. The rind is chartreuse-yellow with
deep longitudinal wrinkles. When ready to eat, the rind is buttery
yellow and the flesh is creamy white, sweet, and without aroma.
It averages four to seven pounds in weight.

Crenshaw. Crenshaw is a hybrid melon, a cross between Persian
and casaba, identified by its large size and distinctive shape
(usually weighing seven to nine pounds). The rind of an immature crenshaw will be green, smooth, with no netting and little
ribbing. As it matures, the skin becomes mottled with yellow and
turns to almost a solid yellow-gold color at the peak of ripeness
and flavor. The flesh is golden-pink, juicy, almost spicy, with a
full aroma.

[1] Based on a two-ounce serving of cooked meat at $3.00/pound of edible raw portion.

Persian. Dark green rind with fine gray netting when ripe. The average size is four to eight pounds with globular-shape fruit. The flesh is orange, very thick, mildly sweet, and has a pleasant aroma when ripe.

Santa Claus or Christmas. Oblong in shape with green and gold rind forming a striped effect. The fruit weighs six to nine pounds and keeps very well in storage. The meat is in shades of green with a mild, slightly sweet flavor.

Canary. The canary melon, first planted in the United States in 1972, is canary yellow and oblong in shape. Flesh is sweet and white with a tinge of pink around the seed cavity. Ripeness is determined by softness at the ends.

Care: Melons require careful handling to prevent damage. Sweetness and flavor of melons does not completely develop until a full-ripe stage of maturity is reached. The total sugar content of the melon does not increase once cut from the vine. Do not expect an immature melon to ripen. Ripeness in almost all melons is indicated by the softening of the fruit surrounding the "eye" or "button" at the blossom end, yielding to gentle pressure of the finger. Most melons diffuse an odor, which becomes stronger and more perceptible when fully ripened. No one indication is infallible; sometimes one, and sometimes a combination of indications must be considered as a guide. Cold storage is not advised. Melons are quickly affected by extremes of either very cold or very hot temperatures. Flavor and texture can be improved if they are held for a few days at 60 °F prior to eating.

Nutrition: Nutritional content varies among the different varieties. The honeydew melon, per 100 grams, will include in its nutritive content, 500 International Units of vitamin A, 32 milligrams of vitamin C, and 41 calories.

Nutritive content of crenshaws and Persians is comparable to that of a cantaloupe and includes 4200 International Units of vitamin A, 45 milligrams of vitamin C, and 31 calories, per 100 grams.

Casabas, Santa Claus, and canary melons have only a trace of vitamin C, and 26 calories.

Generally, the darker the orange color of the meat, the richer it is as a source of vitamin A. All melons are a good source of potassium.

Uses: Melons are delicious by themselves and mixed with other fruits for low-calorie salads. Some good combinations include: sliced peaches and honeydew melon; melon, pineapple, and blueberries or strawberries; bananas and cantaloupe; honeydew melon, blueberries and bananas.

Nectarines

Care: Nectarines, like peaches, do not gain sugar once they have been picked, and must be harvested at maturity. Holding them at room temperature for two to three days is usually enough to complete ripening.

To select a nectarine, look for a creamy yellow background and well-formed fruit without bruises. The crimson blush of nectarines is an indication of variety, not maturity. At ripeness, the fruit will give slightly to gentle palm pressure. Too long storage may cause red to brown discoloration and wooliness in the flesh during the ripening process, even though the exterior may remain normal.

Nutrition: One medium-sized nectarine provides about 45 percent of the RDA of vitamin A and about 30 percent of that for vitamin C. One nectarine contains about 88 calories.

Uses: Nectarines are as versatile as any other fresh fruit, as they complement cereals, poultry dishes, desserts and breads.

Peaches

Care: A bright, fresh appearance is a good clue to a high-quality peach. Background color should be either yellowish or creamy. A greenish color suggests that the peach was immature when picked and will not ripen well. Such a peach will become shriveled or flabby and have tough and poorly flavored skin. The popular red blush may be present on peaches in varying degrees, depending on the variety, but the red color is not a true sign of quality. Peaches that exhibit large flattened bruises will not ripen well. A deep reddish-brown coloring to the fruit or a slight shriveling of the skin at the stem end indicates overripeness.

Nutrition: A medium-size peach contains about 40 calories and provides about 25 percent of the RDA for vitamin A and 10 percent of the vitamin C allowance.

Uses: Peaches are renowned for their use in pies, jams, pancakes, mousses, custards, breads, and souffles.

Pears

Care: Avoid those pears that are prominently bruised, blackened, or that show evidence of punctures or decay, wilting or shriveling. An overripe condition is indicated by obvious softness and discoloration. Scars or other minor skin blemishes generally do not affect the quality of the pear. Russet coloring is a common characteristic among some of the best flavored.

Pears, unlike other fruit are harvested while the skin is still green and the flesh firm, because they won't ripen properly on the tree. Fruit that is allowed to ripen on the tree will develop a coarse, woody or gritty texture. Green pears will ripen for eating by putting them in a loosely closed bag. Keep them together, because pears give off gases that aid each other in ripening.

Nutrition: One medium pear contains trace amounts of the B vitamins, iron, magnesium, and phosphorus, and supplies 12 percent of the RDA of vitamin C.

Uses: Because of their natural sweetness and juiciness, pears are most often enjoyed fresh for snacks. However, new recipes include pears in coffee cakes, with chicken and fish dishes, cooked with liquor (see recipe for Kahlua Pears Meringue on page 261), in quiches, and salads.

For a variety of recipes write to: California Tree Fruit Agreement, P.O. Box 255383, Sacramento, CA 95865.

Prunes

Care: Ready-to-serve prunes come in cans and jars in a variety of sizes and types: *Regular,* packed in syrup; *nectarized,* water-packed with a smaller amount of packing liquid than regular prunes and a higher content of prunes; *high moisture,* a regular dry-pitted prune at a higher moisture level.

Ready-to-use prunes, with pits or pitted, come in transparent bags or in cartons (and sometimes in bulk). Prunes are packed according to size, but pound for pound there is little difference in the amount of edible fruit.[1] Prunes come in four sizes: small, 67 to 85 per pound; medium 53 to 67 per pound; large, 43 to 53 per pound; and extra large, 36 to 43 per pound.

Prunes keep best when stored in a cool, dry place. For long-term storage, keep them in the refrigerator.

Canned or bottled prune juice is also available, and is prepared from a water extract of dried prunes. For best flavor, serve cold.

Nutrition: Prunes are a good addition to your nutritional needs at a moderately low cost. Prunes are especially known for their high iron and potassium contents.

Prunes contain a natural laxative, so far not completely identified chemically, that performs specifically as a regulator of the large intestine. When food intake is low, constipation sometimes develops. Prunes, in addition to foods containing natural fiber (fruits, vegetables, whole grains, legumes, nuts and seeds), are good additions to your diet if you have problems with constipation.

---

[1]Fourteen ounces of pitted prunes is approximately equal to one pound with pits.

Uses: To plump prunes, cover with equal measure of hot or cold water or fruit juice. Refrigerate at least 24 hours. Complementary flavorings include: apple, orange, and pineapple juice; orange or lemon slices; vanilla extract or bean; stick cinnamon; whole cloves or nutmeg. Prunes are a very versatile food and can be incorporated into breads, muffins, cookies, stews, salads, casseroles, cereals, stuffings, soups and puddings to add sweetness and vitamins and minerals.

Spinach

Care: Spinach has a three- to five-day storage life under refrigeration. It should have fresh, crisp, clean leaves, with good green coloring. Plants should be well developed and stocky. Spinach that is straggly, long-stemmed, or overgrown with seed stalks will be undesirable, as will plants with coarse leaf stems, which may be tough. Spinach that is wilted or decayed should be avoided.

Nutrition: Spinach is another nutrient-dense food. One cup of cooked leaves has 41 calories, 5.4 grams of protein and supplies 22 percent of the RDA for iron, 292 percent for vitamin A, 83 percent of vitamin C, and good quantities of thiamine, riboflavin and folacin. Though spinach is sometimes listed as a good source of calcium, it contains a high concentration of oxalic acid, which may interfere with the use of calcium or magnesium present in the diet. Current information is inadequate for determining the extent to which oxalic acid may limit the availability of the various minerals.

Uses: There are many ways in which spinach can be included in your diet. Whether steamed, stir-fried, chopped, creamed, or pureed, it goes nicely as a side dish; in meat loafs, and stuffings; in soups; in quiches; and with rice. The newest and very popular way to serve spinach is raw, as a salad in itself — included in many of our menus.

Tomatoes

Care: Tomato quality is dependent to a large degree upon proper harvesting and handling methods. If a tomato is picked mature when still green, it will ship well and ripen to a good flavor and quality. If it is picked immature, flavor and coloring will suffer. Tomatoes should be plump and well formed, uniform in size and shape and free from bruises.

Most fresh tomatoes sold in supermarkets are firm and not yet ripe. To hasten ripening, place fresh tomatoes in a brown paper bag or in a fruit ripening bowl. As the fruit ripens it emits a natural gas — ethylene. This gas speeds up the ripening process when confined around the fruit in a closed bag or fruit ripening bowl. Allow the fruit to ripen at room temperature, away from direct sunlight. Contrary to popular belief, fresh tomatoes should not be refrigerated before they are fully ripe. Cold temperatures will diminish the flavor, texture and aroma.

Ripe tomatoes should be completely red or reddish-orange, depending on the variety. They will have a sweet, subtle aroma and will give slightly to gentle pressure. Once tomatoes have ripened, they may be kept in the refrigerator for a few days.

Nutrition: A medium-size raw tomato (about 100 grams) contains approximately 20 calories and provides 20 percent of the RDA of vitamin A and 35 percent of the vitamin C allowance. Tomatoes retain vitamin C well with the green fruit, gaining the nutrient as it colors. Tomatoes are also a good source of potassium.

Uses: Tomatoes are a very versatile food. They can be stuffed, stewed, broiled and baked with meats and other vegetables. Of course, they are enjoyed sliced raw into a salad and they make a nice addition to sandwiches, adding moisture when fats (mainly mayonnaise) are limited on low-calorie diets. Tomatoes are widely used in Italian cooking, as a base for many sauces, soups and stews. A pinch of sugar balances the acid and rounds out the flavor of cooked tomato dishes. Because of their high water content, raw tomatoes do not freeze well. However, cooked tomato mixtures may be frozen. For more information and recipes write to: California Fresh Market Tomato Advisory Board, 690 Fifth Street, San Francisco, CA 94107.

Walnuts

Virtually all U.S. walnuts are produced in California. These plantings produce about 45 percent of the world's supply of English walnuts, the most common variety. Other varieties of walnuts are butternuts, black walnuts and hickory nuts.

Care: The care of walnuts in storage is similar to all nuts. See information under *almonds*.

Nutrition: Analysis shows walnuts to contain 67 percent fat, 14.7 percent protein, 12.9 percent carbohydrates, 3.7 percent water, and 1.7 percent minerals.

Vitamins: Walnuts contain trace amounts of vitamin A, riboflavin and niacin, and a one-ounce serving supplies 7 percent of the RDA for thiamine.

Minerals: Walnuts are high in phosphorus and a one-ounce serving supplies 6 percent of the RDA for iron.

Uses: Walnuts used in cooking and bakery products not only tend to fortify food with respect to calories and certain vitamin and mineral values, but add zest and flavor, and give desirable crunchiness to soft foods.

In most instances, walnuts can be added to bread, salads, cookies and muffins with no deviation from standard recipes. They are easy to use and add protein to such lower-priced carbohydrate foods as grains, fruits and vegetables.

For further information contact: Walnut Marketing Board, 155 Bovet Road, San Mateo, CA 94402.

CALIFORNIA'S LEADING FRUITS AND VEGETABLES:
Harvest Season and Importance 1980

Commodity	Harvest Season	National Ranking	California % of U.S. Production	Value ($1000)
Almonds (shelled)	Aug. 5-Oct. 30	1	95	473,340
Apples	July 15-Oct. 30	5	6	40,560
Apricots	June 1-July 25	1	97	32,200
Artichokes	Continuous	1	---	27,473
Asparagus	Feb. 1-June 30	1	47	40,807
Avocados	Nov. 1-Oct. 31	1	73	112,200
Beans, dry	Aug. 20-Nov. 15	2	15	120,006
Beans, green lima	Aug. 15-Oct. 31	1	55	15,785
Beans, snap	Apr. 20-Dec. 15	6	3	12,003
Broccoli	Continuous	1	95	140,178
Brussels sprouts	Aug. 1-Mar. 15	1	--	16,953
Bushberries				
boysenberries	June 1-June 30	--	--	2,386
olallieberries	June 1-Aug. 31	--	--	1,116
raspberries	June 1-July 31	--	--	1,641
Cabbage	Continuous	4	10	12,450
Carrots	Continuous	1	53	94,179
Cauliflower	Continuous	1	75	80,388
Celery		1	63	94,648
central coast	July 1-Dec. 31	--	--	44,008
south coast	Nov. 1-July 31	--	--	50,640
Cherries, sweet	May 20-June 25	2	27	27,676
Corn, sweet	May 1-Dec. 15	9	3	15,076
Cucumbers		4	10	20,282
fresh market	Mar. 20-Nov. 30	--	--	11,610
for pickles	July 1-Sept. 30	--	--	8,672
Dates	Oct. 1-Dec. 15	1	--	13,658
Figs, fresh	June 10-Sept. 15	1	--	12,118
Garlic	Apr. 1-Sept. 15	1	--	35,816
Grapefruit		3	8	22,227
dessert	Nov. 15-July 15	--	--	9,786
other	Mar. 20-Oct. 30	--	--	12,441
Grapes		1	92	1,215,585
raisin type	July 25-Oct. 20	--	--	629,460
table type	July 5-Nov. 5	--	--	164,025
wine type	Sept. 5-Oct. 30	--	--	422,100

Commodity	Harvest Season	National Ranking	California % of U.S. Production	Value ($1000)
Lemons		1	85	136,644
Lettuce		1	74	382,563
winter	Jan. 1-Mar. 31	--	--	63,492
spring	Apr. 1-June 30	--	--	133,540
summer	July 1-Sept. 30	--	--	103,614
fall	Oct. 1-Dec. 31	--	--	81,917
Melons				
cantaloupe	May 15-Nov. 30	1	68	96,338
honeydew	July 10-Nov. 30	1	71	26,316
Persian	June 25-Oct. 31	1	--	1,159
watermelon	May 25-Oct. 15	3	14	26,477
Mushrooms, fresh				
market	Continuous	1	31	73,786
Nectarines	June 15-Aug. 10	1	95	44,468
Olives	Oct. 1-Feb. 15	1	95	38,406
Onions	Apr. 1-Oct. 31	1	28	77,446
Oranges		2	19	224,548
navel and				
miscellaneous	Nov. 1-June 15	--	--	134,638
Valencia	Mar. 15-Dec. 20	--	--	89,910
Peaches		1	66	176,438
Clingstone	July 15-Sept. 15	--	--	129,908
Freestone	May 10-Oct. 5	--	--	46,530
Pears	Aug. 1-Oct. 5	1	45	73,311
Peas, green	Apr. 10-June 10	7	2	2,251
Peppers, bell	July 1-Dec. 10	2	27	18,327
Peppers, chili	Sept. 15-Dec. 15	1	--	12,354
Pistachios	Sept. 15-Dec. 10	1	95	55,760
Plums	May 25-Aug. 30	1	100	71,840
Pomegranates	Sept. 15-Nov. 10	1	95	3,516
Potatoes	Continuous	5	6	157,590
winter	Nov. 20-Apr. 20	2	30	5,076
spring	Apr. 15-Aug. 15	1	51	64,058
summer	June 15-Oct. 15	1	16	30,514
fall	Sept. 10-Mar. 31	11	2	57,942
Prunes, dried basis	Aug. 15-Oct. 30	1	100	112,470
Spinach		1	49	17,881
fresh market	Continuous	1	47	10,684
processing, winter	Mar. 15-May 10	1	50	7,197
Strawberries	Feb. 15-Nov. 30	1	75	201,266
Sweet potatoes	July 15-Nov. 15	3	14	21,726
Tangerines	Nov. 1-May 15	2	23	8,415
Tomatoes		1	79	490,310
fresh market	Apr. 15-Dec. 31	2	29	163,404
processing	June 10-Nov. 10	1	89	326,906
Walnuts	Sept. 25-Oct. 30	1	95	168,300

Source: California Department of Food and Agriculture

PART FOUR:
THE CALIFORNIA DIET
EAT AND PLAY PLANS

Part IV gives you all the information necessary to construct your own, personal California Diet and Exercise Program. In Chapter 3 you will find a detailed explanation of the various components of the program, which are as follows:
- IDEAL WEIGHT TABLE (pages 54 & 55)
  Use this to find your "Ideal Weight."
- MAINTENANCE CALORIE INTAKE TABLE
  Find your Maintenance Calorie Intake from your Ideal Weight.

IDEAL WEIGHT	MAINTENANCE CALORIE INTAKE
(Pounds)	(Low to Moderate Activity)
87-100	1400
101-114	1600
115-126	1800
127-139	2000
140-153	2200
154-166	2400
167-179	2600
180-193	2800

- EAT AND PLAY PLANS
  Find the plan that has a large number corresponding to your Maintenance Calorie Intake. This is your personal guide to eating and playing during your weight-loss year.
- CALORIE PLANS
  These seven-day diets suggest detailed menus to provide appropriate calorie levels of *your* plan, using healthful foods. There are plans for five different daily calorie levels. At the end of each plan is a Nutritional Content Table.
- DAILY FOOD ALLOWANCE
- TYPICAL MEAL PATTERN
  These tables enable you to construct your own menu plans at five different calorie levels, using foods from the Exchange Lists.
- EXCHANGE LISTS
  Use these lists to exchange food items in the Calorie Plans, and to construct your own plans.
- RECIPES
  These are used in the Calorie Plans, and emphasize healthy, California foods.
- PLAY PLANS
  Last but *not* least! These activity plans are essential to successful weight loss, and must be followed together with the Calorie Plans.

THE CALIFORNIA DIET EAT AND PLAY PLANS

1400

ENTRY LEVEL 1400 CALORIES

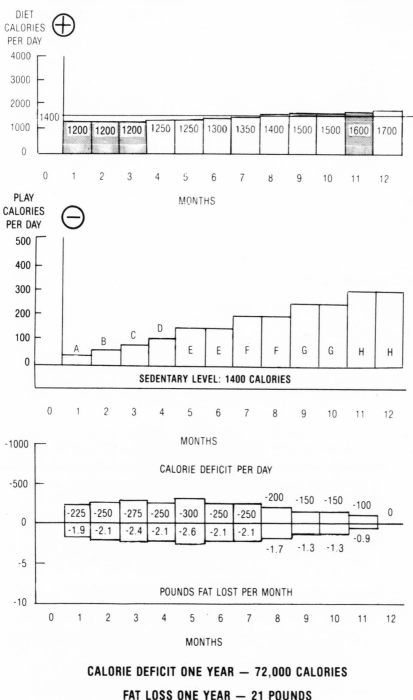

CALORIE DEFICIT ONE YEAR — 72,000 CALORIES

FAT LOSS ONE YEAR — 21 POUNDS

WEIGHT LOSS ONE YEAR — 19 POUNDS

THE CALIFORNIA DIET EAT AND PLAY PLANS

ENTRY LEVEL: 1600 CALORIES

1600

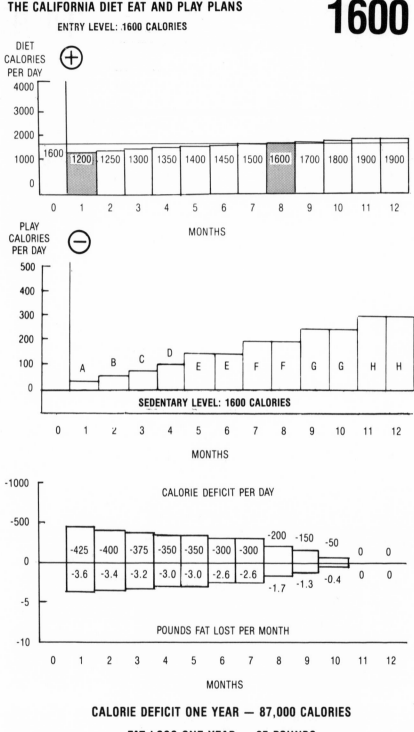

DIET CALORIES PER DAY $\oplus$

4000
3000
2000
1000 · 1600 | 1200 | 1250 | 1300 | 1350 | 1400 | 1450 | 1500 | 1600 | 1700 | 1800 | 1900 | 1900
0

MONTHS

PLAY CALORIES PER DAY $\ominus$

500
400
300
200
100 · A · B · C · D · E · E · F · F · G · G · H · H
0

SEDENTARY LEVEL: 1600 CALORIES

MONTHS

-1000

CALORIE DEFICIT PER DAY

-500

-425 | -400 | -375 | -350 | -350 | -300 | -300 | -200 | -150 | -50 | 0 | 0
-3.6 | -3.4 | -3.2 | -3.0 | -3.0 | -2.6 | -2.6 | -1.7 | -1.3 | -0.4 | 0 | 0

-5

POUNDS FAT LOST PER MONTH

-10

MONTHS

CALORIE DEFICIT ONE YEAR — 87,000 CALORIES

FAT LOSS ONE YEAR — 25 POUNDS

WEIGHT LOSS ONE YEAR — 23 POUNDS

THE CALIFORNIA DIET EAT AND PLAY PLANS

ENTRY LEVEL: 1800 CALORIES

1800

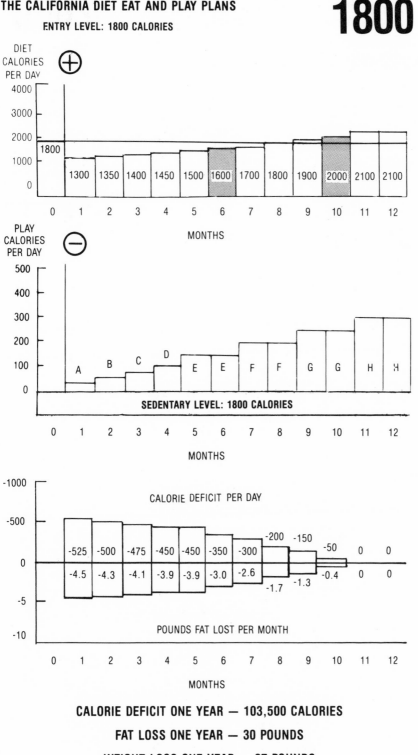

CALORIE DEFICIT ONE YEAR — 103,500 CALORIES

FAT LOSS ONE YEAR — 30 POUNDS

WEIGHT LOSS ONE YEAR — 27 POUNDS

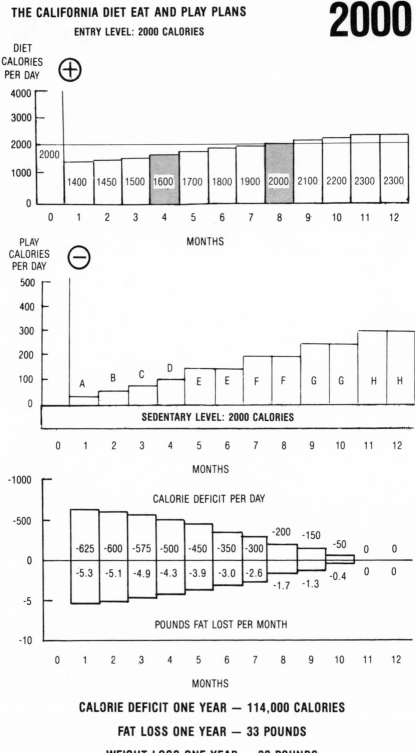

THE CALIFORNIA DIET EAT AND PLAY PLANS

ENTRY LEVEL: 2000 CALORIES

2000

DIET CALORIES PER DAY ⊕

MONTHS

PLAY CALORIES PER DAY ⊖

SEDENTARY LEVEL: 2000 CALORIES

MONTHS

CALORIE DEFICIT PER DAY

POUNDS FAT LOST PER MONTH

MONTHS

CALORIE DEFICIT ONE YEAR — 114,000 CALORIES

FAT LOSS ONE YEAR — 33 POUNDS

WEIGHT LOSS ONE YEAR — 30 POUNDS

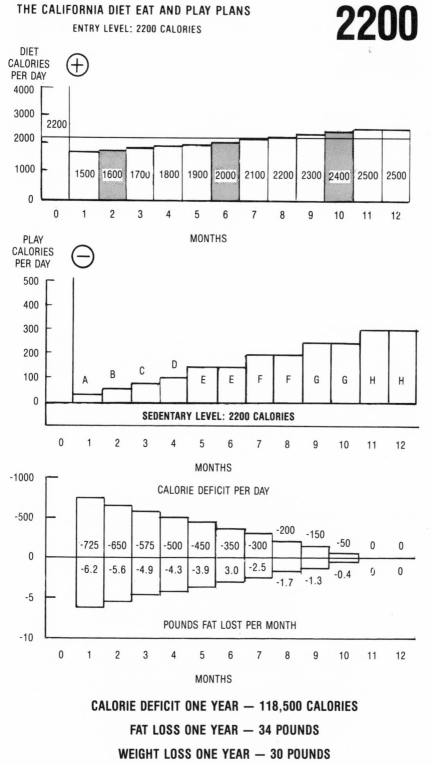

THE CALIFORNIA DIET EAT AND PLAY PLANS
ENTRY LEVEL: 2200 CALORIES

2200

DIET CALORIES PER DAY $\oplus$

4000
3000
2200
2000
1000
0

1500 | 1600 | 1700 | 1800 | 1900 | 2000 | 2100 | 2200 | 2300 | 2400 | 2500 | 2500

0 1 2 3 4 5 6 7 8 9 10 11 12

MONTHS

PLAY CALORIES PER DAY $\ominus$

500
400
300
200
100
0

A B C D E E F F G G H H

SEDENTARY LEVEL: 2200 CALORIES

0 1 2 3 4 5 6 7 8 9 10 11 12

MONTHS

-1000
-500
CALORIE DEFICIT PER DAY
0

-725 | -650 | -575 | -500 | -450 | -350 | -300 | -200 | -150 | -50 | 0 | 0

-6.2 | -5.6 | -4.9 | -4.3 | -3.9 | 3.0 | -2.5 | -1.7 | -1.3 | -0.4 | 0 | 0

-5

POUNDS FAT LOST PER MONTH

-10

0 1 2 3 4 5 6 7 8 9 10 11 12

MONTHS

CALORIE DEFICIT ONE YEAR — 118,500 CALORIES
FAT LOSS ONE YEAR — 34 POUNDS
WEIGHT LOSS ONE YEAR — 30 POUNDS

THE CALIFORNIA DIET EAT AND PLAY PLANS

2400

ENTRY LEVEL: 2400 CALORIES

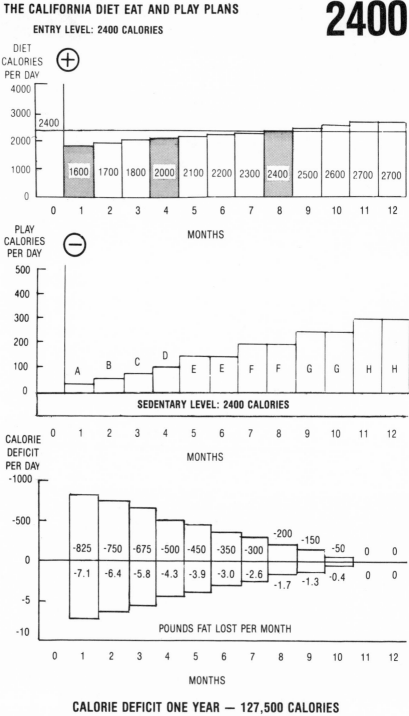

DIET CALORIES PER DAY ⊕

2400

| 1600 | 1700 | 1800 | 2000 | 2100 | 2200 | 2300 | 2400 | 2500 | 2600 | 2700 | 2700 |

MONTHS

PLAY CALORIES PER DAY ⊖

A B C D E E F F G G H H

SEDENTARY LEVEL: 2400 CALORIES

MONTHS

CALORIE DEFICIT PER DAY

| -825 | -750 | -675 | -500 | -450 | -350 | -300 | -200 | -150 | -50 | 0 | 0 |
| -7.1 | -6.4 | -5.8 | -4.3 | -3.9 | -3.0 | -2.6 | -1.7 | -1.3 | -0.4 | 0 | 0 |

POUNDS FAT LOST PER MONTH

MONTHS

CALORIE DEFICIT ONE YEAR — 127,500 CALORIES

FAT LOSS ONE YEAR — 36 POUNDS

WEIGHT LOSS ONE YEAR — 32 POUNDS

200

THE CALIFORNIA DIET EAT AND PLAY PLANS

2600

ENTRY LEVEL: 2600 CALORIES

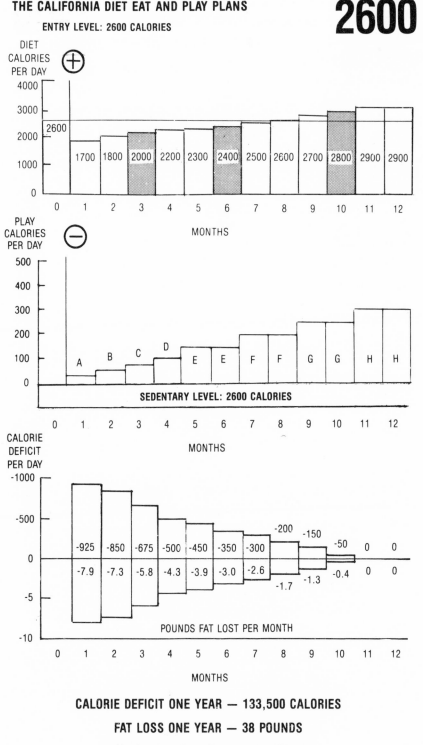

DIET CALORIES PER DAY ⊕

2600

Month	1	2	3	4	5	6	7	8	9	10	11	12
Calories	1700	1800	2000	2200	2300	2400	2500	2600	2700	2800	2900	2900

MONTHS

PLAY CALORIES PER DAY ⊖

A B C D E E F F G G H H

SEDENTARY LEVEL: 2600 CALORIES

MONTHS

CALORIE DEFICIT PER DAY

-925	-850	-675	-500	-450	-350	-300	-200	-150	-50	0	0
-7.9	-7.3	-5.8	-4.3	-3.9	-3.0	-2.6	-1.7	-1.3	-0.4	0	0

POUNDS FAT LOST PER MONTH

MONTHS

CALORIE DEFICIT ONE YEAR — 133,500 CALORIES

FAT LOSS ONE YEAR — 38 POUNDS

WEIGHT LOSS ONE YEAR — 33 POUNDS

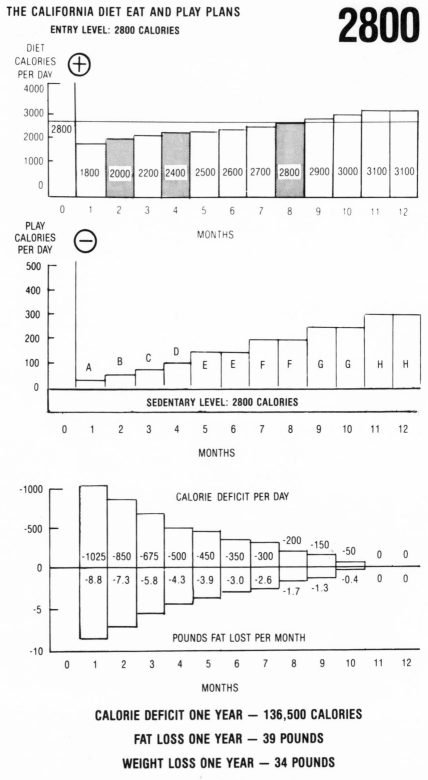

THE CALIFORNIA DIET EAT AND PLAY PLANS

ENTRY LEVEL: 2800 CALORIES

2800

DIET CALORIES PER DAY ⊕

4000
3000
2800
2000
1000
0

| 1800 | 2000 | 2200 | 2400 | 2500 | 2600 | 2700 | 2800 | 2900 | 3000 | 3100 | 3100 |

0   1   2   3   4   5   6   7   8   9   10   11   12

MONTHS

PLAY CALORIES PER DAY ⊖

500
400
300
200
100
0

A   B   C   D   E   E   F   F   G   G   H   H

SEDENTARY LEVEL: 2800 CALORIES

0   1   2   3   4   5   6   7   8   9   10   11   12

MONTHS

-1000

-500

CALORIE DEFICIT PER DAY

| -1025 | -850 | -675 | -500 | -450 | -350 | -300 | -200 | -150 | -50 | 0 | 0 |
| -8.8 | -7.3 | -5.8 | -4.3 | -3.9 | -3.0 | -2.6 | -1.7 | -1.3 | -0.4 | 0 | 0 |

0

-5

POUNDS FAT LOST PER MONTH

-10

0   1   2   3   4   5   6   7   8   9   10   11   12

MONTHS

CALORIE DEFICIT ONE YEAR — 136,500 CALORIES

FAT LOSS ONE YEAR — 39 POUNDS

WEIGHT LOSS ONE YEAR — 34 POUNDS

1200 CALORIE PLAN

SAMPLE MENUS — BASED ON EXCHANGE LISTS

DAY 1

BREAKFAST Orange juice, ½ cup (D); Non-fat milk, 1 cup (Al); whole grain cereal, cooked, ½ cup (E) with 2 tablespoons raisins (D) and 7 almonds (H)

LUNCH Non-fat milk, 1 cup (Al); Sandwich: whole grain bread, 2 slices (E), skim milk cheese, 2 ounces (F1); Salad: spinach, 1 cup (B) with ½ tablespoon dressing (H); Cantaloupe, ¼ (6-inch) (D)

DINNER Chinese beef with vegetables® , 1 serving; Rice, cooked, ½ cup (E); Lettuce salad, 1 cup (B) with 2 tablespoons low-calorie dressing®

DAY 2

BREAKFAST Grapefruit juice, ½ cup (D); Shredded wheat biscuit, 1 (E) with 1 cup non-fat milk (A1) and ½ banana (D); Coffee (I) with 2 tablespoons liquid non-dairy creamer (H)

LUNCH Lentil soup, ¾ cup (G1); Hamburger: lean ground beef, 2 ounces (F1) with 1 slice tomato, lettuce (B), on 1 hamburger bun (E) with 1 teaspoon mayonnaise (H); Non-fat milk, 1 cup (A1); Peach, dried, ½ (D)

DINNER Baked halibut® , 1 serving; Crookneck squash, ½ cup (B); Lettuce salad, 1 cup (B) with 2 tablespoons low-calorie dressing® ; Bran muffin, 1 (2-inch diameter) (E)

DAY 3

BREAKFAST Ready-to-eat cereal (iron fortified), ¾ cup (E) with 1 cup strawberries (D) and 1 cup non-fat milk (A1); Dried apricots, 4 halves (D); Coffee (I) with 2 tablespoons liquid non-dairy creamer (H)

® Recipe included

LUNCH   Grape and ham salad®, 1 serving; Whole wheat bread, 2 slices (E); Non-fat milk, 1 cup (A1)

DINNER   Roast veal, 3 ounces (F1); Baked potato, 1 small (E) with 1 teaspoon margarine (H); Brussels sprouts, cooked, ½ cup (B); Swiss chard salad, 1 cup (B) with ¾ cup kidney beans, cooked (G1) and 2 tablespoons low-calorie dressing®

DAY 4

BREAKFAST Cantaloupe, ¼ (6-inch) and 2 medium prunes (D); Non-fat milk, 1 cup (A1); Rye toast, 1 slice (E) with 1 teaspoon margarine (H)

LUNCH   Bean-beef enchilada®, 2; Spinach, cooked, ½ cup (B); Non-fat milk, 1 cup (A1); Fig, dried, 1 small (D)

DINNER   Roast chicken, 3 ounces (F1); Brown rice, cooked, ½ cup (E); Summer squash, ½ cup (B); Watercress salad, 1 cup (B) with ½ tablespoon dressing (H)

DAY 5

BREAKFAST Prune juice, ¼ cup (D); Skim milk, 1 cup (A1); 1 tangerine (D); Whole wheat toast, 1 slice (E) with 1 teaspoon peanut butter (H)

LUNCH   Cold chicken salad: chicken cooked, diced, 2 ounces (F1), bulgar wheat, cooked ⅓ cup (E), tomato, cucumber, diced, ¼ cup each (B) on a bed of lettuce (B) with 2 tablespoons low-calorie dressing®; Non-fat milk, 1 cup (A1); Whole wheat bread, 1 slice (E) with 1 teaspoon margarine (H); Molded fruit salad®, 1 serving

DINNER   Taco: taco shell 1 (E, H)*; lean ground beef, 3 ounces (F1); Pinto beans, cooked, ¾ cup (G1); Lettuce, tomato, ¼ cup each (B); Lettuce salad, 1 cup (B) with broccoli, ½ cup (B) and 2 tablespoons low-calorie dressing®

---

*Pre-made taco shells contain about one fat exchange. If homemade, you may fry in one teaspoon oil.

DAY 6

BREAKFAST	Grapefruit, ½ (D); Cream of wheat, cooked, ½ cup (E) with 2 tablespoons raisins (D); Non-fat milk, 1 cup (A1); Coffee (I) with 2 tablespoons liquid non-dairy creamer (H)
LUNCH	Non-fat milk, 1 cup (A1); Tofu quiche®, 1 serving; Endive salad, 1 cup (B) with 2 table-spoons low-calorie dressing® ; Boston brown bread, 1 slice (E); Blueberries, ½ cup (D)
DINNER	Cod, broiled, 3 ounces (F1) with lemon, herbs (I); Corn, ⅓ cup (E); Broccoli, steamed, ½ cup (B) with 1 teaspoon margarine (H)

DAY 7

BREAKFAST	Fruit salad: Dates, 2 small (D), orange, sec-tioned, ½ (D), almonds, slivered, 1 tablespoon (H), topped with ½ cup evaporated non-fat milk (A1); Whole wheat muffin, 1 (2-inch) (E)
LUNCH	Burrito: flour tortilla, 1 (6-inch) (E), lean ground beef, 2 ounces (F1), 1 tablespoon sour cream (H), spices (I), lettuce, ½ cup, tomato, 1 slice (B); Skim milk, 1 cup (A1); Blackberries, ½ cup (D) and 1 slice whole wheat bread (E)
DINNER	Black bean soup, ¾ cup (G1); Coq au Vin®, 1 serving; Noodles, cooked, ½ cup (E); Aspara-gus, ½ cup (B); Spinach, 1 cup and mush-rooms, ½ cup, salad (B) with 2 tablespoons low-calorie dressing®

1200 CALORIE PLAN

NUTRITIONAL CONTENT

(AVERAGE DAILY INTAKE OVER SEVEN DAYS OF PLAN)

CALORIES	1232
PROTEIN (grams)	87
TOTAL FAT (grams)	27
TOTAL CARBOHYDRATES (grams)	160
% PROTEIN CALORIES	28
% FAT CALORIES	20
% CARBOHYDRATE CALORIES	52
POLYUNSATURATED/SATURATED FAT (P/S) RATIO	1.08
REFINED SUGAR (grams)	1
NATURAL SIMPLE SUGARS (grams)	75
STARCH (grams)	77
CHOLESTEROL (milligrams)	151
CALCIUM (milligrams)	1007
PHOSPHORUS (milligrams)	1472
MAGNESIUM (milligrams)	352
IRON (milligrams)	17
ZINC (milligrams)	13
VITAMIN A (International units)	12,203
THIAMINE (milligrams)	1.3
RIBOFLAVIN (milligrams)	2.2
NIACIN (milligrams)	20
VITAMIN C (milligrams)	180
VITAMIN B_6 (milligrams)	2.1
FOLACIN (micrograms)	285

1200 CALORIE PLAN

DAILY FOOD ALLOWANCE

FOOD GROUP	NUMBER OF SERVINGS	CHOOSE FROM LIST
Milk	2	A1
Vegetables	2-4	B
Fruits	3	D
Bread	4	E
Protein Foods		
Animal	5	F1
Vegetable	1	G1, 2
Fats	3	H
Free Foods	As Desired (AD)	I

TYPICAL MEAL PATTERN

BREAKFAST
1 Serving Milk (A1)
2 Servings Fruit (D)
1 Serving Bread (E)
1 Serving Fat (H)

LUNCH
1 Serving Milk (A1)
At least 1 Serving Vegetable (B)
1 Serving Fruit (D)
2 Servings Bread (E)
2 Servings Animal Protein (F1)
1 Serving Vegetable Protein (G1, 2) (or at dinner)
1 Serving Fat (H)

DINNER
At least 1 Serving Vegetable (B)
1 Serving Bread (E)
3 Servings Animal Protein (F1)
1 Serving Vegetable Protein (G1, 2) (or at lunch)
1 Serving Fat (H)

SNACK
AD Free Foods (I)

SAMPLE MENUS — BASED ON EXCHANGE LISTS

DAY 1

BREAKFAST	Non-fat milk, 1 cup (A1); Oatmeal, cooked, 1 cup (E) with 2 teaspoons margarine (H); Honey-dew melon, ¼ (7-inch diameter) (D)
LUNCH	Non-fat milk, 1 cup (A1); Tuna sandwich: water- packed tuna, 2 ounces (F1) with 2 teaspoons mayonnaise (H), whole grain bread, 2 slices (E); Spinach, ½ cup, cooked (B); Tangerine, 1 (D)
DINNER	Ragout of Beef with marjoram® , 1 serving; Lettuce salad, 1 cup (B) with ¾ cup garbanzo beans, cooked (G1) and 1 tablespoon salad dressing (H); Whole wheat bread, 1 slice (E)
SNACK	Raisins, 2 tablespoons (D)

DAY 2

BREAKFAST	Banana milkshake® ; Whole grain cereal, 1 cup, cooked (E) with 2 tablespoons sunflower seeds (H)
LUNCH	Non-fat milk, 1 cup (A1); Lentil soup, ¾ cup (G1); Endive salad, 1 cup (B) with 2 ounces skim milk cheese, grated (F1) and 1 tablespoon salad dressing (H); Melba toast, 2 (E); Peach, dried, ½ (D)
DINNER	Pork shank, 3 ounces (F1) with ½ cup tomato juice (C); Mashed potatoes, ½ cup (E); Green peas, ½ cup (C); Swiss chard salad, 1 cup (B) with 1 tablespoon dressing (H); Gingersnaps, 2 (E)
SNACK	Orange juice, ½ cup (D)

® Recipe included

DAY 3

BREAKFAST Banana, ½ and strawberries, 1 cup, sliced (D) with ½ cup evaporated non-fat milk (A1); Whole wheat toast, 2 slices (E) with 2 teaspoons margarine (H)

LUNCH Sandwich: turkey, 2 ounces (F1), whole wheat bread, 2 slices (E), tomato, lettuce (B); Non-fat milk, 1 cup (A1) ; Salad: lentils, ¾ cup, cooked (G1), 6 walnut halves (H), with 2 table-spoons low-calorie dressing® on lettuce bed (B); Pear, 1 small (D)

DINNER Pasta Alla Piemontese® , 1 serving; Romaine lettuce salad, 1 cup, with radishes and cucum-bers (B) and ½ tablespoon dressing (H)

SNACK Prunes, 2 medium (D)

DAY 4

BREAKFAST Orange sections, 1 small (D); Whole grain toast, 1 slice (E); with 2 teaspoons peanut butter (H); Non-fat milk, 1 cup (A1); Ready-to-eat cereal, iron fortified, ¾ cup (E)

LUNCH Pea and turnip bisque® , 1 serving; Cornbread (1½-inch cube) (E); Chili: ¾ cup pinto beans, cooked (G1), 2 ounces lean ground beef (F1), spices (I); Shredded cabbage salad, 1 cup (B) with 2 tablespoons low-calorie dressing® and 2 tablespoons raisins (D)

DINNER Cornish Hen, roasted, 3 ounces (F1); Brown rice, ½ cup, cooked (E); Mustard greens, ½ cup (B), sauteed with 1 teaspoon oil (H); Muffin, 1 (2-inch diameter) (E) with 1 teaspoon margarine (H); Carrot sticks, raw, 1 cup (C)

SNACK Grapes, 12 (D)

DAY 5

BREAKFAST Prune juice, ½ cup (D); Non-fat milk, 1 cup (A1); Eggs, poached, 2 (F2 from lunch) on 2 toasted English muffin halves (E) with 2 tea-spoons margarine (H)

LUNCH	Non-fat milk, 1 cup (A1); Bean burrito® , 1 serving; Brown rice, ½ cup, cooked (E); Escarole salad, 1 cup, with radishes and red pepper (B); 1 tablespoon salad dressing (H); Molded fruit salad® , 1 serving
DINNER	Broiled cod, 3 ounces (F1) with lemon and herbs (I); Corn, 2 small ears (E) with 2 teaspoons margarine (H); Acorn squash, 1 cup (C)
SNACK	Grapefruit, ½ (D)

DAY 6

BREAKFAST	Bran flakes, 1 cup (E) with ½ banana (D) and 1 cup non-fat milk (A1); Tangerine, 1 sliced (D) with ¼ cup liquid non-dairy creamer (H)
LUNCH	Lettuce salad, 1 cup (B) with 2 ounces shrimp (F1); ¾ cup dried white beans, cooked (G1) and 2 tablespoons low-calorie dressing® ; Bagel, 1 (E) with 2 teaspoons margarine (H); Casaba, diced, 1 cup (D); Non-fat milk, 1 cup (A1)
DINNER	Chilled, cooked artichoke, 4 ounces (C) with 2 tablespoons low-calorie dressing® ; Chicken Pilau® , 1 serving; ½ cup cubed butternut squash (C) with 1 teaspoon margarine (H)
SNACK	Apricots, dried, 4 halves (D)

DAY 7

BREAKFAST	Grapefruit juice, ½ cup (D); Non-fat milk, 1 cup (F1); Whole wheat pancakes, 2 (E) with ½ cup blueberries (D) and 2 teaspoons margarine (H)
LUNCH	Non-fat milk, 1 cup (A1); Stir fry: sliced chicken, 2 ounces white meat (F1), peapods, ½ cup, Chinese greens, ½ cup (B) in 2 teaspoons oil (H) and ½ tablespoon cornstarch (E) and ½ cup broth (I); Enriched white rice, cooked, 1 cup (E); Fig, dried, 1 (D)

DINNER   Veal shank, 3 ounces (F1) in ½ cup tomato
juice (C) with onions, 2 tablespoons, garlic, and
celery, (B); Noodles, 1 cup (E); Bean and carrot
vinaigrette® , 1 serving on a bed of lettuce (B)

SNACK   Cherries, 10 (D)

1600 CALORIE PLAN

NUTRITIONAL CONTENT

(AVERAGE DAILY INTAKE OVER SEVEN DAYS OF PLAN)

CALORIES	1556
PROTEIN (grams)	93
TOTAL FAT (grams)	44
TOTAL CARBOHYDRATES (grams)	199
% PROTEIN CALORIES	24
% FAT CALORIES	25
% CARBOHYDRATE CALORIES	51
POLYUNSATURATED/SATURATED FAT (P/S) RATIO	1.58
REFINED SUGAR (grams)	2
NATURAL SIMPLE SUGARS (grams)	87
STARCH (grams)	102
CHOLESTEROL (milligrams)	220
CALCIUM (milligrams)	1025
PHOSPHORUS (milligrams)	1555
MAGNESIUM (milligrams)	443
IRON (milligrams)	19
ZINC (milligrams)	15
VITAMIN A (International units)	12,698
THIAMINE (milligrams)	2.1
RIBOFLAVIN (milligrams)	2.3
NIACIN (milligrams)	23
VITAMIN C (milligrams)	161
VITAMIN B_6 (milligrams)	2.5
FOLACIN (micrograms)	390

1600 CALORIE PLAN

DAILY FOOD ALLOWANCE

FOOD GROUP	NUMBER OF SERVINGS	CHOOSE FROM LIST
Milk	2	A1
Vegetables		
Low calorie	2-4	B
Moderate calorie	2	C
Fruits	4	D
Bread	6	E
Protein Foods		
Animal	5	F1
Vegetable	1	G1, 2
Fats	6	H
Free Foods	As Desired (AD)	I

TYPICAL MEAL PATTERN

BREAKFAST
1 Serving Milk (A1)
2 Servings Fruit (D)
2 Servings Bread (E)
2 Servings Fat (H)

LUNCH
1 Serving Milk (A1)
At least 1 Serving Vegetable (B)
1 Serving Fruit (D)
2 Servings Bread (E)
2 Servings Animal Protein (F1)
1 Serving Vegetable Protein (G1, 2) (or at dinner)
2 Servings Fat (H)

DINNER
At least 1 Serving Vegetable (B)
2 Servings Vegetable (C)
2 Servings Bread (E)
3 Servings Animal Protein (F1)
1 Serving Vegetable Protein (G1, 2) (or at lunch)
2 Servings Fat (H)

SNACK
1 Serving Fruit (D)
AD Free Foods (I)

2000

SAMPLE MENUS — BASED ON EXCHANGE LISTS

DAY 1

BREAKFAST
Orange juice, ½ cup (D); Bran flakes, 1 cup (E) with ½ banana, sliced (D) and 1 cup low-fat milk (A2); Whole wheat toast, 1 slice (E) with 2 teaspoons peanut butter (H)

LUNCH
Creamy cucumber soup®, 1 serving; Taco (2): 2 corn tortillas* (6-inch) (E), each fried in 1 teaspoon oil (H), 2 ounces lean ground beef (F1), ¾ cup cooked pinto beans (G1) with 2 tablespoons onion, ¼ cup tomato and 1 cup shredded lettuce (B); Apricots, dried, 4 halves (D); Fig, dried, 1 (D); Low-fat milk, 1 cup (A2)

DINNER
Snapper, 3 ounces, broiled (F1); Spinach, ½ cup (B); Pumpkin squash, whipped, 1 cup (C); Lettuce salad, 1 cup (B) with ½ tablespoon dressing (H); Dinner rolls, 2 (2-inch diameter) (E) with 2 teaspoons margarine (H)

SNACK
sponge cake, 2, 1½ inch cube (E), topped with 1 cup blueberries (D)

DAY 2

BREAKFAST
Banana milkshake® made with low-fat milk (A2) and 3 tablespoons wheat germ (E); Whole wheat toast, 2 slices (E) with 2 teaspoons margarine (H)

LUNCH
Grilled cheese sandwich: whole wheat bread, 2 slices (E), with 2 ounces skim milk cheese (F1) and 1 slice tomato (B); Low-fat milk, 1 cup (A2); Tangerine, 2 small (D)

DINNER
Baked chicken, 3 ounces white meat (F1); Rice with chili®, 1 serving; Carrots, ½ cup cooked (C); Spinach salad, 1 cup (B) with ½ tablespoon

® Recipe included

*If pre-made taco shell is used, it already contains one serving of fat.

dressing (H); Whole wheat bread, 1 slice (E) with 1 teaspoon margarine (H)

SNACK   Plain bagel, 1 (E) with 1 tablespoon margarine (H from lunch); 1 small apple, and prunes, 2 medium (D)

DAY 3

BREAKFAST   Grapefruit juice, ½ cup (D); Low-fat milk yogurt (A2) with 1 medium peach, sliced (D); Oatmeal, 1 cup, cooked (E) with 2 tablespoons liquid non-dairy creamer (H); Whole wheat bread, 1 slice (E) with 1 teaspoon margarine (H)

LUNCH   Low-fat milk, 1 cup (A2); Cod, 2 ounces, baked (F1); Noodles, 1 cup cooked (E) with parsley, 2 tablespoons (B); Asparagus, ½ cup (B); Apple and endive salad®, 1 serving; Plum, 2 medium (D)

DINNER   Leg of lamb, 3 ounces, roasted (F1); Brown rice, 1 cup cooked (E) with 6 whole pecans, chopped (H); Acorn squash, 1 cup, cubed (C); Tossed green salad, 1 cup (B) with ¾ cup kidney beans, cooked (G1) and 2 tablespoons low-calorie dressing®

SNACK   Apricot nectar, ⅔ cup (D); Bran muffin, 2 (2-inch diameter) (E)

DAY 4

BREAKFAST   Prune juice, ¼ cup (D); Iron-fortified, ready-to-eat cereal, 1½ cups (E) with ½ cup rasp-berries (D); Low-fat milk, 1 cup (A2); Blueberry whole wheat muffin, 1 (2-inch) (E) with 1 tea-spoon margarine (H); Coffee (I) with 2 table-spoons liquid non-dairy creamer (H)

LUNCH   Low-fat milk, 1 cup (A2); Chicken sandwich: whole wheat bread, 2 slices (E), chicken, 2 ounces white meat, cooked, chopped (F1), mayonnaise, 1 tablespoon (H); Broccoli, cooked, ½ cup (B) with 1 teaspoon lemon (I); Nectarine, 1 medium (D)

DINNER	Split pea soup, ¾ cup (G1); Lemon sole® , 1 serving; Carrots, 1 cup, julienne (C) with ½ cup zucchini steamed (B); New potatoes, 2 small boiled (E); Butter lettuce salad, 1 cup (B) with 1 tablespoon dressing (H)
SNACK	Pineapple juice, ⅔ cup (D); Graham crackers, 4 (2½ inch square) (E)

DAY 5

BREAKFAST	Grapefruit juice, 1 cup (D); Low-fat milk, 1 cup (A2); Eggs, 2 poached (F2 from lunch); Hash browns, 1 cup shredded potatoes (E) fried in 1 teaspoon oil (H); Whole wheat toast, 1 slice (E) with 1 teaspoon margarine (H)
LUNCH	Sandwich: whole wheat bread, 2 slices (E), tofu, grilled, 4 ounces (G2), 1 teaspoon mayonnaise (H), 1 slice tomato (B); Low-fat milk, 1 cup (A2); Coleslaw: cabbage, 1 cup shredded (B), 1 tablespoon dressing (H); Banana, 1 (D)
DINNER	Turkey, 3 ounces, roasted, white meat (F1); Bulgur wheat, ⅓ cup, cooked (E); Broccoli A L'Orange® , 1 serving; Acorn squash, 1 cup (C), topped with 3 tablespoons bread crumbs (E) and 2 teaspoons margarine (H)
SNACK	Cornbread, 2 (1½ inch cube) (E); Apple, 1 medium (D)

DAY 6

BREAKFAST	Stewed prunes, 4 (D); Cream of wheat, 1 cup, cooked (E); Low-fat milk, 1 cup (A2); Whole wheat muffin, 1 (2-inch) (E) with 2 teaspoons margarine (H)
LUNCH	Chef salad: lettuce, 1 cup (B), garbanzo beans, ¾ cup cooked (G1), radishes, cucumber, tomatoes, green pepper, celery, 1 cup total (B); salad dressing, 1 tablespoon (H); Whole wheat bread, 1 slice (E); Low-fat milk, 1 cup (A2); Lemon-pineapple cheese pie® , 1 serving; Fig, dried, 1 (D)

DINNER	Tomato juice, 1 cup (C); Roast veal, 3 ounces (F1); Baked potato, 1 medium (E) with 2 tablespoons sour cream (H); Green beans, ½ cup (B)
SNACK	Melba toast, 2 slices (E); Pear, 1 medium (D)

DAY 7

BREAKFAST	Orange juice, ½ cup (D); Whole wheat pancakes, 3 (4-inch) (E) with ½ cup blueberries (D) and 2 teaspoons margarine (H); Low-fat milk, 1 cup (A2)
LUNCH	Black bean soup, ¾ cup (G1); Lean pork, 2 ounces (F1); Yam, ¼ cup (E) with 1 teaspoon margarine (H); Cabbage and apple slaw® , 1 serving; Whole wheat bread, 1 slice (E) with 1 teaspoon margarine (H); Plum, 2 medium (D)
DINNER	Broiled chicken, 3 ounces (F1) with herbs (I); ½ cup Brussels sprouts (B); Brown rice, ½ cup, cooked (E); Beet salad, 1 cup sliced (C) with 1 tablespoon vinaigrette dressing (H); Dinner roll (2-inch) 1 small (E) with 1 teaspoon margarine (H)
SNACK	Low-fat milk yogurt, 1 cup (A2 from lunch) with 2 medium prunes, chopped, and apricots, dried, 4 halves, chopped (D); Plain muffins, 2 (2-inch diameter) (E)

2000 CALORIE PLAN

NUTRITIONAL CONTENT

(AVERAGE DAILY INTAKE OVER SEVEN DAYS OF PLAN)

CALORIES	2032
PROTEIN (grams)	98
TOTAL FAT (grams)	65
TOTAL CARBOHYDRATES (grams)	263
% PROTEIN CALORIES	19
% FAT CALORIES	29
% CARBOHYDRATE CALORIES	52

POLYUNSATURATED/SATURATED FAT (P/S) RATIO	1.05
REFINED SUGAR (grams)	10
NATURAL SIMPLE SUGARS (grams)	119
STARCH (grams)	125
CHOLESTEROL (milligrams)	261
CALCIUM (milligrams)	1143
PHOSPHORUS (milligrams)	1731
MAGNESIUM (milligrams)	507
IRON (milligrams)	20
ZINC (milligrams)	17
VITAMIN A (International units)	16,534
THIAMINE (milligrams)	1.9
RIBOFLAVIN (milligrams)	2.7
NIACIN (milligrams)	25
VITAMIN C (milligrams)	195
VITAMIN B_6 (milligrams)	2.8
FOLACIN (micrograms)	418

2000 CALORIE PLAN

DAILY FOOD ALLOWANCE

FOOD GROUP	NUMBER OF SERVINGS	CHOOSE FROM LIST
Milk	2	A2
Vegetables		
Low-calorie	2-4	B
Moderate calorie	2	C
Fruits	6	D
Bread	9	E
Protein Foods		
Animal	5	F1
Vegetable	1	G1, 2
Fats	8	H
Free Foods	As Desired (AD)	I

TYPICAL MEAL PATTERN

BREAKFAST
1 Serving Milk (A2)
2 Servings Fruit (D)
3 Servings Bread (E)
2 Servings Fat (H)

LUNCH
1 Serving Milk (A2)
At least 1 Serving Vegetable (B)
2 Servings Fruit (D)
2 Servings Bread (E)
2 Servings Animal Protein (F1)
1 Serving Vegetable Protein (G1, 2) (or at dinner)
3 Servings Fat (H)

DINNER
At least 1 Serving Vegetable (B)
2 Servings Vegetable (C)
2 Servings Bread (E)
3 Servings Animal Protein (F1)
1 Serving Vegetable Protein (G1, 2) (or at lunch)
3 Servings Fat (H)

SNACK
2 Servings Fruit (D)
2 Servings Bread (E)
AD Free Foods (I)

SAMPLE MENUS — BASED ON EXCHANGE LISTS

DAY 1

BREAKFAST	Orange juice, ½ cup (D); Honeydew melon, ¼ (7-inch diameter) (D); Iron-fortified, ready-to-eat cereal, ¾ cup (E); Low-fat milk, 1 cup (A2); Whole wheat toast, 2 slices (E) with 2 teaspoons peanut butter (H); Coffee (I) with 2 tablespoons liquid non-dairy creamer (H).
LUNCH	Fish chowder®, 1 serving (contains 1 vegetable "C" from dinner and 1 milk "A2" from snack); Tofu sandwich: 2 slices whole wheat bread (E), 4 ounces grilled tofu (G2) with 1 slice tomato (B); Dried prunes, 4 medium (D)
DINNER	Lamb chop, 3 ounces, broiled (F1); Applesauce, ½ cup, unsweetened (D); Mashed potatoes, 1 cup (E); Fresh peas, ½ cup (C); Lettuce salad, 1 cup (B) and 1 tablespoon salad dressing (H); Dinner roll, 1 (2-inch diameter) (E) with 1 teaspoon margarine (H)
SNACK	Sponge cake 2 (1½ inch cube) (E) with 2 medium peaches, sliced (D)

DAY 2

BREAKFAST	Grapefruit juice, 1 cup, unsweetened (D); Oatmeal, 1 cup, cooked (E) with 2 tablespoons raisins (D); Low-fat milk, 1 cup (A2); English muffin, ½ (E) with 2 teaspoons margarine (H); Coffee (I) with 2 tablespoons liquid non-dairy creamer (H)
LUNCH	Chicken enchilada: 1 flour tortilla, 6-inch (E), 2 ounces shredded chicken, cooked (F1), ½ cup tomato juice (B) with 1 tablespoon onion, chopped (B), pinto beans, ¾ cup, cooked (G1); Brown rice, 1 cup, cooked (E) with 2 teaspoons margarine (H); Spinach, ½ cup, cooked (B); with 1 teaspoon margarine (H); Apple, 1 medium (D)

® Recipe included

DINNER   Veal stew: 3 ounces lean veal, cubed (F1), ½ cup carrots, cooked (C), noodles, 1 cup, cooked (E); Salad: ½ cup sliced cucumbers (B) and ½ cup sliced tomatoes (C) with 1 tablespoon salad dressing (H); Saltine crackers, 3 (2-inch square) (E); Apricot-almond tapioca® , 1 serving

SNACK   low-fat yogurt, 1 cup (A2), with 1 banana, sliced (D), 2 (2-inch) blueberry muffins (E)

DAY 3

BREAKFAST   Grape juice, ¾ cup, unsweetened (D); Cream of wheat, 1 cup, cooked (E) with 2 teaspoons margarine (H); Low-fat milk, 1 cup (A2); Whole wheat toast, 1 slice (E) with 1 teaspoon margarine (H)

LUNCH   Tuna-bean salad® , 1 serving; French roll, 3 ounces (E); Fruit salad: 12 grapes and ½ cup mandarin oranges, (unsweetened) (D)

DINNER   Apple juice, ⅓ cup (D); Chateaubriand, 3 ounces, broiled (F2); Baked potato, 1 medium (E) with 2 teaspoons margarine (H); Eggplant casserole: ½ cup eggplant (B), with ½ cup tomato sauce (C), topped with 3 tablespoons bread crumbs (E); Chilled, cooked, artichoke, 4 ounces (C) with ½ tablespoon vinaigrette salad dressing (H)

SNACK   bran flakes cereal, 1 cup (E) with 1 medium nectarine, sliced (D) and 1 cup low-fat milk (A2)

DAY 4

BREAKFAST   Orange juice, 1 cup (D); French toast: 3 slices whole wheat bread (E), 2 eggs (F2 from lunch), 1 tablespoon oil (H), top with ½ cup crushed pineapple (D); Low-fat milk, 1 cup (A2)

LUNCH   Lentil soup, ¾ cup (G1); Soda crackers, 6 (2½ inch square) (E); Spinach salad: 1 cup spinach (B), ½ cup mushrooms, sliced (B) with 1 tablespoon dressing (H); Rye bread, 1 slice (E) with 1 teaspoon margarine (H); Baked apple, 1 medium (D)

DINNER   Curried chicken® , 1 serving; White enriched rice, 1 cup, cooked (E); Cubed winter squash, 1 cup (C); Strawberry crepes: 2 (6-inch) crepes® (E) each filled with ½ cup strawberries sliced (D), topped with 2 tablespoons sour cream (H)

SNACK   Low-fat yogurt, 1 cup (A2) with 1 medium peach, sliced (D) and 2 dates, chopped (D); Whole wheat bread, 1 slice (E); 3 cups popcorn, unbuttered (E)

DAY 5

BREAKFAST   Prune juice, ½ cup (D); Shredded wheat, 2 biscuits (E) with banana, ½ sliced (D); Low-fat milk, 1 cup (A2); Whole wheat toast, 1 slice (E) with 2 teaspoons margarine (H); Coffee (I) with 2 tablespoons liquid non-dairy creamer (H)

LUNCH   California salad: 1 cup lettuce (B) , ½ cup low-fat cottage cheese (F1), ¾ cup garbanzo beans, cooked (G1), honeydew melon, 1/8 (7-inch diameter), sliced (D), plums, 2 medium, sliced (D), avocado, 1/8 (4-inch diameter) (H) with 1 tablespoon salad dressing (H); Melba toast, 3 slices (E)

DINNER   Poached salmon, 3 ounces (F2); Fresh peas, ½ cup (C); Lemon potatoes with dill® , 1 serving; Salad: 4 ounces tomatoes (C), sliced with 2 tablespoons onion, sliced (B), avocado 1/8 (4-inch diameter) (H) with ½ tablespoon dressing (H); Whole wheat bread, 2 slices (E); Molded fruit salad® , 1 serving

SNACK   Tapioca: made with 1 cup low-fat milk (A2), 4 tablespoons tapioca (E), 1 cup crushed pine-apple (D)

DAY 6

BREAKFAST   Grapefruit, ½ (D); Whole grain cereal, 1 cup, cooked (E) with 4 tablespoons raisins (D) and 7 almonds, chopped (H); Low-fat milk, 1 cup (A2); Whole wheat toast, 1 slice (E)

LUNCH   Navy bean soup, ¾ cup (G1); Roast chicken, 2 ounces white meat, cooked (F1); Brown rice, 1 cup, cooked (E) with 6 walnut halves, chopped (H); Spinach, ½ cup, cooked (B); Whole wheat bread, 1 slice (E) with 1 teaspoon margarine (H); Figs, 2 small, dried (D)

DINNER   Pasta Alla Piemontese® , 1 serving; Salad: Romaine lettuce, 1 cup (B), 1 tablespoon dressing (H); French bread, 1 ounce or 1 slice (E); Watermelon, 1 cup, diced (D)

SNACK   Raspberry-honey muffin® , 1 (contains 2 fat exchanges from breakfast) (H); Low-fat milk, 1 cup (A2); Vanilla wafers, 3 (E); Peach, 1 medium (D)

DAY 7

BREAKFAST   Orange juice, 1 cup, unsweetened (D); Buttermilk pancakes, 3 (5 × ½ inch) (E) with ½ cup applesauce, unsweetened (D); and 3 teaspoons margarine (H); 1 cup low-fat yogurt (A2)

LUNCH   Chicken chop suey: 2 ounces chicken, diced (F1), 4 ounces tofu, diced (G2), ¼ cup chopped celery (B), ¼ cup sliced mushrooms (B), ½ cup bean sprouts (B), ½ cup noodles, cooked (E), all sauteed in 1 tablespoon oil (H); 1 cup steamed white rice (E); Sliced pineapple, 1 cup (D)

DINNER   Onion soup, 1 cup (C) with 1 slice toasted bread (E) and 1 ounce melted skim milk cheese (F2); 1 cup lettuce (B) with ½ tablespoon salad dressing (H); Whole wheat bread, 2 slices (E) with 2 teaspoons margarine (H); Orange cheese souffle® , 1 serving; Raspberries, ½ cup (D)

SNACK   Cornbread, 2, 1½ inch cubes (E); 1 cup low-fat milk (A2); 4 fresh figs (D)

2400 CALORIE PLAN

NUTRITIONAL CONTENT

(AVERAGE DAILY INTAKE OVER SEVEN DAYS OF PLAN)

CALORIES	2375
PROTEIN (grams)	106
TOTAL FAT (grams)	74
TOTAL CARBOHYDRATES (grams)	322
% PROTEIN CALORIES	18
% FAT CALORIES	28
% CARBOHYDRATE CALORIES	54
POLYUNSATURATED/SATURATED FAT (P/S) RATIO	1.16
REFINED SUGAR (grams)	7
NATURAL SIMPLE SUGARS (grams)	146
STARCH (grams)	160
CHOLESTEROL (milligrams)	312
CALCIUM (milligrams)	1206
PHOSPHORUS (milligrams)	1781
MAGNESIUM (milligrams)	558
IRON (milligrams)	22
ZINC (milligrams)	18
VITAMIN A (International units)	12,637
THIAMINE (milligrams)	2.0
RIBOFLAVIN (milligrams)	2.7
NIACIN (milligrams)	27
VITAMIN C (milligrams)	186
VITAMIN B_6 (milligrams)	3.1
FOLACIN (micrograms)	440

2400 CALORIE PLAN

DAILY FOOD ALLOWANCE

FOOD GROUP	NUMBER OF SERVINGS	CHOOSE FROM LIST
Milk	2	A2
Vegetables		
Low-calorie	2-4	B
Moderate calorie	2	C
Fruits	8	D
Bread	11	E
Protein Foods		
Animal	5	F1, 2
Vegetable	1	G1, 2
Fats	9	H
Free Foods	As Desired (AD)	I

TYPICAL MEAL PATTERN

BREAKFAST
1 Serving Milk (A2)
3 Servings Fruit (D)
3 Servings Bread (E)
3 Servings Fat (H)

LUNCH
At least 1 Serving Vegetable (B)
2 Servings Fruit (D)
3 Servings Bread (E)
2 Servings Animal Protein (F1, 2)
1 Serving Vegetable Protein (G1, 2) (or at dinner)
3 Servings Fat (H)

DINNER
At least 1 Serving Vegetable (B)
2 Servings Vegetable (C)
1 Serving Fruit (D)
3 Servings Bread (E)
3 Servings Animal Protein (F1, 2)
1 Serving Vegetable Protein (G1, 2) (or at lunch)
3 Servings Fat (H)

SNACK
1 Serving Milk (A2)
2 Servings Fruit (D)
2 Servings Bread (E)
AD Free Foods (I)

SAMPLE MENUS — BASED ON EXCHANGE LISTS

DAY 1

BREAKFAST   Orange juice, ½ cup (D); Bran flakes, 1 cup (E) with 2 tablespoons raisins (D); Low-fat milk, 1 cup (A2); Whole wheat bread, 1 slice (E) with 1 tablespoon peanut butter (H); Coffee (I) with 2 tablespoons liquid, non-dairy creamer (H)

LUNCH   Low-fat milk, 1 cup (A2); Chicken and hazel nut salad®, 1 serving; Melba toast, 3 slices (E); Carrot sticks, 1 cup (C); Pear, medium, 1 (D)

DINNER   Apple juice, ⅔ cup (D); Swiss steak, 3 ounces (F1) with 2½ tablespoons flour (E), ½ cup to-mato juice (C), ½ cup onion (C) and 1 tea-spoon oil (H); Noodles, cooked, 1 cup (E); Spinach salad, 1 cup (B) and 1 tablespoon dress-ing (H); Dinner roll, 1 (2-inch) (E)

SNACK   Fig bar cookies, 3 (E), Apple juice, ⅔ cup, nectarine, 1 medium, (D), walnut halves, 6 (H)

DAY 2

BREAKFAST   Fruit salad: 1 cup diced mixed fruit (D) topped with 1 cup low-fat yogurt (A2), 7 almonds, 3 walnut halves (H) and 3 tablespoons wheat germ (E); Whole wheat bread, 2 slices (E) with 2 tea-spoons margarine (H)

LUNCH   Tomato juice, 1 cup (C); Stuffed bellpepper: 1 pepper (B), 2 ounces ground lean beef (F1), ½ cup cooked enriched white rice (E); Pita bread ½ (E) with spread: ¾ cup cooked, ground, garbanzo beans (G1), 1 tablespoon sesame but-ter (H), spices and lemon juice, 1 teaspoon (I); Low-fat yogurt, ½ cup (A2) with 4 small dates, diced (D)

® Recipe included

DINNER	Coquilles-Saint Jacques® , 1 serving (contains ½ cup milk exchange "A2" from lunch); Saffron white rice, 1 cup, cooked (E); Green peas, 1 cup (C); Butter lettuce salad, 1 cup (B) with ½ tablespoon dressing (H); French bread, 2 slices (E); Raspberries, 1 cup (D), with 2 tablespoons non-dairy creamer (H)
SNACK	Granola, ½ cup (E, H) with 4 tablespoons raisins (D); orange juice, 1 cup (D); Popcorn, 3 cups, unbuttered (E)

DAY 3

BREAKFAST	Grapefruit juice, 1 cup (D); Cream of wheat, 1 cup (E), cooked, with 1 cup low-fat milk (A2); Topped with ¼ cup liquid non-dairy creamer (H); Whole wheat toast, 1 slice (E) with 2 teaspoons margarine (H)
LUNCH	Cantaloupe, ½, sliced (D), with 1 ounce proscuito (F1); Dinner roll, 2 (2-inch) (E); Spinach crepe, 2: crepes® 2, each filled with ¼ cup spinach, cooked (B) and part skim ricotta cheese, 1 ounce (F2); Sauce: 3 teaspoons margarine (H), 1 teaspoon flour (E), ½ cup evaporated low-fat milk (A2); Acorn squash, 1 cup, cubed (C)
DINNER	Chicken stew: 3 ounces chicken (F1), lima beans, ¾ cup, cooked (G1), red potatoes, 2 small (E), corn, ⅓ cup (E), tomato paste, ¼ cup (C); Swiss chard salad, 1 cup (B) with 1 orange, sectioned (D), and 1 tablespoon dressing (H); Whole wheat bread, 1 slice (E) with 1 teaspoon margarine (H)
SNACK	Graham cracker, 4 (2½ inch square) (E); Oatmeal cookies® , 2; grape juice, ¾ cup (D)

DAY 4

BREAKFAST	Orange juice, ½ cup (D); Strawberry waffles: 3 waffles (5 × ½ inch) (E) with 1 cup strawberries (D), 3 teaspoons margarine (H), topped with 1 cup low-fat yogurt (A2); Coffee (I) with 2 tablespoons liquid non-dairy creamer (H)

LUNCH	Louie salad: 1 cup lettuce (B), 2 ounces crab (F1), ¼ (4-inch diameter) avocado, sliced (H), honeydew melon, ¼ (7-inch diameter) sliced (D) with 2 tablespoons low-calorie dressing® ; Tamale pie: pinto beans, ¾ cup, cooked (G1), onion, ½ cup (C), tomato paste, 2 tablespoons (C), corn, ⅓ cup (E), cornmeal, 1 cup, cooked (E), olives, 5 small, black (H); 1 cup low-fat milk (A2)
DINNER	Tomato juice, ½ cup (C); Lamb and vegetables with lime® , 1 serving; White rice, ½ cup, cooked (E) with ¼ cup raisins (D) and 7 almonds, chopped (H); Sweet potato, ¾ cup, baked (E) with 2 teaspoons margarine (H); Broccoli, ½ cup, steamed (B)
SNACK	Pineapple juice, 1 cup (D); Lemon meringue pie (¹/₈ of 9-inch) [2 fat (H), 1 fruit (D), 2 bread (E)]; plain muffin, 1 (2-inch) (E)

DAY 5

BREAKFAST	Banana milkshake® (made with low-fat milk); Add 3 tablespoons wheat germ (E); Plain muffin, 1 (2-inch) (E) with 1 teaspoon margarine (H); Ready-to-eat cereal, iron fortified, ¾ cup (E) with 6 tablespoons liquid non-dairy creamer (H)
LUNCH	Low-fat milk, 1 cup (A2); Mushroom-rice salad with pine nuts® , 1 serving; Chicken, 2 ounces, roasted (F1); Potato, 1 medium, oven brown (E); Beets, 1 cup, steamed (C); Orange, 1 (D)
DINNER	Beef burgundy: 3 ounces lean beef, cubed (F1), ½ cup each carrots and onions (C), mushrooms, ¼ cup (B), garlic, herbs (I); wine, 4 ounces (used in cooking) (I); Noodles, 1 cup, cooked (E) with 1 teaspoon margarine (H); Lettuce salad, 1 cup (B) with 2 tablespoons low-calorie dressing® ; Whole wheat bread, 2 slices (E) with 2 teaspoons margarine (H); Pear, 1 medium (D)
SNACK	Melba toast, 3 slices (E) with 2 teaspoons margarine (H); Prune juice, ½ cup (D); 1 medium apple (D)

DAY 6

BREAKFAST Cantaloupe, ½ (D); Omelet: 2 eggs [(F2) from lunch]; Hash browns: 2 small potatoes, shredded (E), cooked in 3 teaspoons oil (H); Whole wheat toast, 1 slice (E) with 1 teaspoon margarine (H); Low-fat milk, 1 cup (A2)

LUNCH Lima bean casserole® , 1 serving; White rice, 1 cup, cooked (E); Spinach salad, 1 cup (B) with 1 cup sliced tomatoes (C) and 1 tablespoon dressing (H); Rye crackers, 3 (E); Pear, 1 medium (D)

DINNER Sea bass, 3 ounces, poached (F1) with parsley and lemon, 1 teaspoon each (I); Julienne vegetables, steamed: 1 cup carrots (C) and ½ cup zucchini (B); Scalloped potatoes: 1 medium potato, sliced (E) with sauce: 1 teaspoon margarine (H), 1 teaspoon flour (E), ½ cup evaporated low-fat milk (A2 from lunch); Dinner roll, 2 small (E) with 2 teaspoons margarine (H); Fruit compote: ½ cup blueberries and 1 medium peach, sliced (D)

SNACK Peach crepes® , 2; Plain muffins, 2 (2-inch) (E); Grapefruit juice, 1 cup (D)

DAY 7

BREAKFAST Low-fat yogurt, 1 cup (A2) with 1 tablespoon sunflower seeds (H) and 1 orange sectioned (D); Whole grain toast, 1 slice (E) with 1 tablespoon peanut butter (H); Oatmeal 1 cup, cooked (E)

LUNCH Grilled cheese sandwich: whole wheat bread, 2 slices (E), 1 teaspoon mayonnaise (H), 2 ounces farmers cheese (F1); Low-fat milk, 1 cup (A2); Tossed salad: 1 cup lettuce (B), 1 cup diced beets (C), ¾ cup kidney beans, cooked (G1) with 1 tablespoon dressing (H); Melba toast, 1 slice (E); Apple, 1 medium (D)

DINNER Chinese soup: Scallions, 1 ounce (B), ½ cup Chinese greens (B) cooked in 1 cup clear broth (I); Sweet and sour chicken: 3 ounces chicken, white meat, cubed, cooked (F1), 1 tablespoon oil (H), 4 ounces pineapple chunks (D) with ⅓

cup pineapple juice, unsweetened (D), ½ cup
carrots (C), ½ cup green onion (C), 1 ounce
green pepper (B), 2 tablespoons cornstarch (E),
1 tablespoon vinegar (I), clear broth, ½ cup (I);
White rice, steamed, 1½ cups, cooked (E)

SNACK   Kahlua Pears Meringue® , 1 serving; Plain
bagel, 1 (E) with 2 teaspoons margarine (H);
Gingersnaps, 2 small (E)

2800 CALORIE PLAN

NUTRITIONAL CONTENT

(AVERAGE DAILY INTAKE OVER SEVEN DAYS OF PLAN)

CALORIES	2799
PROTEIN (grams)	111
TOTAL FAT (grams)	87
TOTAL CARBOHYDRATES (grams)	393
% PROTEIN CALORIES	16
% FAT CALORIES	28
% CARBOHYDRATE CALORIES	56
POLYUNSATURATED/SATURATED FAT (P/S) RATIO	1.14
REFINED SUGAR (grams)	11
NATURAL SIMPLE SUGARS (grams)	190
STARCH (grams)	178
CHOLESTEROL (milligrams)	279
CALCIUM (milligrams)	1291
PHOSPHORUS (milligrams)	2007
MAGNESIUM (milligrams)	661
IRON (milligrams)	27
ZINC (milligrams)	20
VITAMIN A (International units)	23,546
THIAMINE (milligrams)	2.5
RIBOFLAVIN (milligrams)	3.3
NIACIN (milligrams)	31
VITAMIN C (milligrams)	343
VITAMIN B_6 (milligrams)	3.8
FOLACIN (micrograms)	550

2800 CALORIE PLAN

DAILY FOOD ALLOWANCE

FOOD GROUP	NUMBER OF SERVINGS	CHOOSE FROM LIST
Milk	2	A2
Vegetables		
Low calorie	2-4	B
Moderate calorie	4	C
Fruits	10	D
Bread	13	E
Protein Foods		
Animal	5	F1, 2
Vegetable	1	G1, 2, 3
Fats	12	H
Free Foods	As Desired (AD)	I

TYPICAL MEAL PATTERN

BREAKFAST
1 Serving Milk (A2)
2 Servings Fruit (D)
3 Servings Bread (E)
4 Servings Fat (H)

LUNCH
1 Servings Milk (A2)
At least 1 Serving Vegetable (B)
2 Servings Vegetable (C)
2 Servings Fruit (D)
3 Servings Bread (E)
2 Servings Animal Protein (F1, 2)
1 Serving Vegetable Protein (G1, 2, 3) (or at dinner)
3 Servings Fat (H)

DINNER
At least 1 Serving Vegetable (B)
2 Servings Vegetable (C)
2 Servings Fruit (D)
4 Servings Bread (E)
3 Servings Animal Protein (F1, 2)
1 Serving Vegetable Protein (G1, 2, 3) (or at lunch)
3 Servings Fat (H)

SNACK
4 Servings Fruit (D)
3 Servings Bread (E)
2 Servings Fat(H)

A. MILK EXCHANGE

A1. Non-Fat	Serving Size	Grams
(Each serving = 80 calories)		
Skim milk	1 cup	240
Powdered (non-fat, dry)	¼ cup	35
Buttermilk made from skim milk	1 cup	240
Canned, evaporated-skim milk	½ cup	120
Yogurt made from skim milk (plain)	1 cup	240
A2. Low-Fat		
(Each serving = 120 calories)		
Low-fat milk (2% fat)	1 cup	240
Yogurt made from 2% fat milk)	1 cup	240
A3. Whole Milk		
(Each serving = 160 calories)		
Whole milk	1 cup	240
Canned, evaporated whole milk	½ cup	120
Powdered milk (whole, dry)	¼ cup	35
Buttermilk made from whole milk	1 cup	240
Yogurt made from whole milk (plain)	1 cup	240

This list shows the kinds and amounts of milk or milk products to use for one Milk Exchange. Adults as well as children need the nutrients found in milk, particularly calcium and riboflavin. It is also a good source of protein, phosphorus, vitamins A, B_{12}, and, if fortified, vitamin D.

If you are unable to eat milk products, it is important to substitute other foods that are rich in calcium such as blackstrap molasses, sunflower and sesame seeds, bok choy, kale, mustard greens, broccoli, asparagus, okra, tofu, dandelion greens, dry beans, soy beans, cabbage, rutabagas, turnips, carrots, dates, figs, oranges and whole wheat bread. Calcium is important for the health of bones, teeth and muscles.

B/C. VEGETABLE EXCHANGE

B. Low Calorie
A serving equals 1 cup raw or ½ cup cooked (unless otherwise indicated). One exchange of most vegetables on this list is approximately 25 calories or less.

Asparagus
Bamboo shoots
Bean sprouts
Beans, green or wax
Broccoli[1]
Brussels sprouts[1]
Cabbage
Cauliflower
Celery
Chicory
Chinese cabbage
Chives
Cucumbers
Eggplant
Endive
Escarole
Fennel

Greens:[1]
  Beet
  Chards
  Collards
  Dandelion
  Kale
  Mustard
  Spinach
  Turnip
Jicama root
Lettuce
Mushrooms
Okra
Onion (1 slice)
Parsley
Pea pods
Peppers, green or red
Radishes

Rhubarb
  (unsweetened)
Sauerkraut
Scallions
Squash (summer)
  Casserta
  Chayote
  Cymling
  Pattypan
  Scalloped
  Spaghetti
  Straight or
    Crookneck
  Zucchini
Tomatoes (limited
  to ½ cup or 1
  medium
Watercress[1]
Wintermelon

Raw celery, chicory, chives, chinese cabbage, cucumbers, endive, escarole, lettuce, parsley and watercress can be used as desired.

[1]Select one dark green leafy vegetable every day.

C. Moderate Calorie.
A serving equals ½ cup. One exchange of most vegetables on this list is approximately 50 calories.[1]

Artichoke
Beets
Carrots
Kohlrabi
Onions
Parsnips

Pumpkin
Rutabaga
Squash (winter)
  Acorn
  Banana
  Butternut

Danish
Des Moines
Hubbard
Tomato juice
Tomato paste
  (¼ cup)
Turnips

[1]One bread exchange may be substituted for two "C" vegetable exchanges without a substantial change in calories, and carbohydrate and protein content.

Each type of vegetable makes a somewhat different contribution to your diet. Dark green and deep yellow are among the leading sources of vitamin A. Some vegetables such as asparagus, broccoli, Brussels sprouts, cauliflower, cabbage, green pepper, greens and tomatoes contain vitamin C. Green leafy vegetables contain iron, folacin, vitamin B_6, potassium, zinc and magnesium. Try to include *at least one serving* of dark-green leafy vegetables in your diet each day. Vegetables are good sources of fiber. Canned vegetable products contain an appreciable amount of sodium unless indicated as low sodium.

D. FRUIT EXCHANGE

Each serving (fresh, dried, cooked, canned, frozen without added sugar) contains 50 calories.

Item	Serving Size	Grams
Apple, fresh	1 small (2-inch diameter)	80
Apple, dried	½ ounce	15
Apple juice	⅓ cup	80
Applesauce, unsweetened	½ cup	100
Apricots, fresh	2 medium	100
Apricots, dried	4 halves	20
Apricot nectar	⅓ cup	80
Banana	½ small	50
Berries[1]		
Blackberries	½ cup	75
Blueberries	½ cup	75
Boysenberries	½ cup	75
Raspberries	½ cup	75
Strawberries	1 cup	150
Cherries	10 large	75
Cider	⅓ cup	80
Cranberries, cooked	1 cup unsweet-ened, chopped	270
Cranberry juice cocktail	¼ cup	60
Dates	2 small	15
Figs, fresh	2	50
Figs, dried	1 small	15
Fruit cocktail	½ cup (drained)	100
Grapefruit[1]	½	125
Grapefruit juice[1]	½ cup	100
Grapes	12 large	75
Grape juice	¼ cup	60
Guava	½ medium	60
Kiwi	1	60
Kumquat	3 medium	60
Lemon juice[1]	¾ cup	180
Loquat	6	100
Mandarin orange[1]	½ cup	100
Mango[1]	½ small	70
Melons[1]		
Cantaloupe	¼ (6-inch)	200
Casaba	1 cup, diced	170

Item	Serving Size	Grams
Honeydew	1/8 (7-inch diameter)	150
Watermelon	1 cup, cubed	175
Nectarine	½ medium (2½-inch)	100
Orange[1]	½ medium	125
Orange juice[1]	½ cup	100
Papaya[1]	⅓ medium	150
Passion fruit	3	100
Peach, fresh	1 medium (2¾-inch)	100
Peach, dried	½ ounce	15
Peach nectar	⅓ cup	80
Pear, fresh	1 small	100
Pear, dried	½ ounce	15
Pear nectar	⅓ cup	80
Persimmon		
Japanese, kaki	⅓ (2½-inch diameter × 3-inch)	70
Native	1	40
Pineapple	½ cup	80
Pineapple juice	⅓ cup	80
Plums	2 medium	100
Pomegranate	1 (2½-inch × 2½-inch)	120
Prunes, dried	2 medium	25
Prune juice	¼ cup	60
Raisins	2 tablespoons	15
Tangelo[1]	1 medium	170
Tangerine[1]	1 medium	100

All fruits contribute fiber and nutrients to your diet, but in different quantities. Vitamin C is abundant in citrus fruits, melons and berries. Try to include *at least one serving* of citrus fruit in your diet each day (or a vegetable source that is high in vitamin C, see Vegetable Exchange). The better sources of vitamin A are those fruits that are orange in color, i.e., dried apricots, mangoes, cantaloupes, papaya, nectarines, peaches and persimmons. Many fruits are valuable sources of folacin (cantaloupes, oranges, strawberries) and potassium (bananas, oranges, plums, dried fruits).

[1]Select one vitamin C-rich fruit every day.

E. BREAD EXCHANGE
(Includes bread, cereal and other starches)
(One serving = 100 calories)

Item	Serving Size	Grams
Bread and rolls		
Bread		
French	1 slice	25
Pumpernickel	1 slice	25
Rye	1 slice	25
White	1 slice	25
Whole wheat	1 slice	25
Bread cubes, dry	½ cup	25
Bread crumbs, dry	3 table-spoons	25
Biscuit (omit 1 fat exchange)	1 (2-inch diameter)	35
Boston brown	1 slice	35
Bagel	½	30
Cornbread (omit 1 fat exchange)	1½-inch cube	35
Corn muffin (omit 1 fat exchange)	1 (2-inch diameter	35
Hamburger bun	½	30
Hot dog bun	½	30
Muffin (omit 1 fat exchange)	1 (2-inch diameter	35
Muffin, English	½	35
Pita bread	¼ (7-inch diameter)	22
Roll, dinner	1 (2-inch diameter)	35
Taco Shell (omit 1 fat exchange)	1	30
Tortilla, flour, corn	1 (6-inch diameter)	30
Cereals		
Bran flakes	½ cup	25
Cereal, cooked	½ cup	100
Cereal, puffed (unfrosted)	1 cup	15
Cereal, ready-to-eat, unsweetened	¾ cup	20
Cornmeal, dry	2 table-spoons	20
Granola (omit 1 fat exchange)[1]	¼ cup	30

Item	Serving Size	Grams
Crackers[2]		
Arrowroot	3	20
Graham	2 (2½-inch square	20
Matzoth	½ (4-inch × 6-inch diameter)	20
Melba toast	1 slice	20
Oyster	20 (⅓ cup)	20
Pretzels	25 (3⅛-inch long × ⅛-inch diameter)	20
Round, thin	6-8 (1½-inch diameter	20
Rye wafers	3 (2-inch × 3½-inch)	20
Saltines	6 (2-inch square)	20
Soda	4 (2½-inch square)	20
Other Grains and Starches		
Barley, cooked	½ cup	100
Bulgur wheat, cooked	⅓ cup	45
Corn	⅓ cup or 1 small ear	80
Crepe	1 (6-inch diameter)	30
Millet, cooked	½ cup	100
Pancake	1 (5-inch × ½-inch)	30
Pasta (cooked)		
Noodles	½ cup	100
Macaroni	½ cup	100
Spaghetti	½ cup	100
Potato		
French fries (omit 1 fat exchange)	8 (3-inch length)	40
Sweet or Yams	¼ cup	50
White (baked, boiled)	1 small	100
White (mashed)	½ cup	100
Popcorn (no butter)	3 cups	20

Item	Serving Size	Grams
Rice (cooked)	½ cup	100
Waffle	1 (5-inch × 4-inch × ½-inch)	30
Wheat bran	4 tablespoons	15
Wheat germ	3 tablespoons	20
Miscellaneous		
Cake, angel food or sponge (no icing)	1½-inch cube	25
Cookies		
Arrowroot	4	20
Fig bar	1	20
Gingersnap	2	20
Vanilla wafers	3	20
Cornstarch	2 tablespoons	20
Flour	2½ tablespoons	20
Potato or corn chips[2] (omit 2 fat exchanges)	15	20
Tapioca	2 tablespoons	20

---

[1]Amount of fat varies considerably with manufacturer. Check label for calorie content.
[2]Items may be high in sodium.

Complex carbohydrates (starches) are often lacking in "fad" diets. Contrary to popular misconception, eating starches does not automatically lead to weight gain. It is a question of how much is eaten and what is eaten with them (i.e., high-fat foods such as butter or margarine, sour cream, etc.). Whole grain and enriched breads and cereals are important sources of thiamine, riboflavin, niacin, iron, vitamin B_6, magnesium, zinc and folacin. The whole grain, bran, and germ products have more fiber than products made from refined flours. Quick breads, such as muffins, biscuits and corn bread, have more fat than most yeast breads. Before making your choice, check the ingredient label or the recipe for added salt, sugar or fat.

F/G. PROTEIN EXCHANGE

ANIMAL PRODUCTS		Serving Size[1]	Grams
F1. Lean Meat			
(Serving = 55 calories) (less than 10% fat)			
Beef:	Baby beef, chipped beef[3], chuck flank steak, tenderloin, plate ribs, plate skirt steak, round, rump, sirloin, tripe, shank	1 ounce	30
Lamb:	Leg, rib, sirloin, loin (roast and chops), shank, shoulder	1 ounce	30
Pork:	Leg (whole rump, center shank); ham[3], smoked[3]	1 ounce	30
Veal:	Leg, loin, rib, shank, shoulder, cutlets	1 ounce	30
Poultry:	Meat without skin of chicken, turkey, cornish hen, guinea hen, pheasant, rabbit	1 ounce	30
Fish:[2]	Cod, flounder, haddock, halibut, perch, sea bass, sole, tuna canned in water[3], abalone, crayfish, octopus, scallops, shrimp, squid, turtle, catfish, smelts, sturgeon, fresh tuna, clams, crab, lobster, mussels, oysters, schrod	1 ounce	30
Cheeses containing less than 5% butterfat[3]		1 ounce	30
Cottage cheese, dry curd and 2% butterfat[3]		¼ cup	60

F2. Medium Fat
(Serving = 75 calories) (15% fat)

Beef:	Ground (15% fat) corned beef[3] (canned), rib eye, round	1 ounce	30

F/G. PROTEIN EXCHANGE

ANIMAL PRODUCTS F2. Medium Fat		Serving Size[1]	Grams
Pork:	Loin (all cuts), tenderloin, shoulder arm, shoulder blade (Boston butt), Canadian bacon[3], boiled ham[3], picnic ham[3], pigs feet[3]	1 ounce	30
Liver, heart, kidney and sweetbreads (these are high in cholesterol)		1 ounce	30
Egg[4] (high in cholesterol)		1	50
Fish:[2]	Albacore, carp, salmon, tuna (canned in oil, drained)[3]	1 ounce	30
Cheese:[3]	Cottage cheese, creamed	¼ cup	60
	Ricotta part-skim	¼ cup	60
	Part-skim mozzarella, Neufchatel, farmer's cheese	1 ounce	30

F3. High Fat
(Serving = 100 calories) (more than 20% fat)

Beef:	Brisket, corned beef [3](Brisket), ground beef (more than 20% fat), chuck (ground commercial), roasts (rib), steaks (club and rib); Pastrami[3]	1 ounce	30
Lamb:	Breast	1 ounce	30
Pork:	Spare ribs, loin (back ribs), ground, country style ham[3], deviled ham[3], bacon[3], salt pork[3]	1 ounce	30
Veal:	Breast	1 ounce	30
Poultry:	Capon, duck (domestic), goose	1 ounce	30
Fish:[2]	Anchovies, herring, mackeral, sardines, shad, trout, tuna (canned in oil)[3], eel	1 ounce	30
Cheeses:[3]	Whole milk ricotta	¼ cup	60
	Cheddar, cream, gruyere, brick, jack, Swiss, American, blue, feta, parmesan, romano, brie, colby,	1 ounce	30

F/G. PROTEIN EXCHANGE

ANIMAL PRODUCTS	Serving Size[1]	Grams
F3. High Fat		
gjetost, muenster, port-salut, Roquefort, Cheshire, processed cheese spread, provolone, gouda, limburger, edam, camembert, tilsit, whole milk mozzarella	1 ounce	30
Cold cuts[3]	1 (4½ × 1/8-inch slice)	30
Frankfurter[3]	1 (4½ × ¾-inch)	30
Sausages[3]	1 ounce	30
Salami[3]	1 ounce	30

[1]Three-ounce serving of cooked meat is about equal to 4 ounces of raw meat.
[2]From American Heart Association, Alameda County Chapter, California.
[3]Items are high in sodium.
[4]Limit to 2 to 3 per week.

The menus offer a variety of choices from this group. The important thing is to select and prepare these foods to moderate the amount of fat. To do so, select lean cuts of meat, trim off the visible fat, and remove skin and fat from poultry. It is also important to moderate the use of salted meats. Canned, dried or pickled meats are high in sodium. Organ meats and egg yolks are sources of many nutrients, but they are also well supplied with cholesterol. Meat, fish, and poultry products are valued sources of protein, phosphorus, vitamins B_6 and B_{12}, iron and zinc. To plan a diet low in saturated fat and cholesterol, choose those exchanges in Lean Meat.

VEGETABLE PRODUCTS[7]	Serving Size[1]	Grams
G1. Low Fat		
(Serving = 150 calories)[2]		
Dried beans, peas (cooked, drained) includes kidney, lima, navy, pinto, split peas, black-eyed peas, lentils, garbanzo, red, pink, black, broad, cow peas, mung, white	¾ cup	140
Soups (bean, pea, lentil)	¾ cup	180
G2. Medium Fat		
(Serving = 100 calories)[3]		
Soybeans (cooked)	½ cup	90
Tofu	4 ounces	120

G3. High Fat

	Serving Size	Grams
(Serving = 200 calories) (omit 2 fat exchanges)		
Nuts, seeds[4, 5]	1 ounce	30
Peanut butter[6]	2 table-spoons	30

In addition to the starch they contribute, dried beans, peas and nuts are generally good sources of protein, iron, zinc, magnesium, phosphorus, thiamine, vitamin B_6, and folacin. These foods, as distinct from animal sources of protein, do not contain vitamin B_{12} (present only in foods of animal origin). These protein sources also contain fiber. Protein foods of plant origin have *no cholesterol*.

---

[1]Based on Modification of the Basic Four Food Guide. *Journal of Nutrition Education* Vol. 10 No. 1 pp. 27-9, Jan-Mar 1978.

[2]Protein = 10 grams, fat = 1 gram.

[3]Protein = 10 grams, fat = 5 grams.

[4]Average of sunflower seeds and peanuts.

[5]Protein = 7 grams, fat = 14 grams.

[6]Protein = 8 grams, fat = 8 grams.

[7]If legumes (dried beans and peas) are not desired in your diet, 2 meat exchanges (beef, lamb, pork, veal, poultry or fish) may be substituted for each serving of legumes without reducing nutrient content substantially. Canned vegetable products contain appreciable amounts of sodium unless indicated as low sodium.

H. FAT EXCHANGE

(50 Calories)

Polyunsaturated Fat	Serving Size	Grams
Mayonnaise[1]	1 teaspoon	5
Oil	1 teaspoon	5
Corn		
Cottonseed		
Safflower		
Soybean		
Sunflower		
Wheat germ		
Salad Dressing[1]		
Clear type (oil and vinegar), regular	½ table-spoon	10
Clear type (oil and vinegar), low-calorie	3 table-spoons[2]	45
Mayonnaise type, regular	½ table-spoon	10
Mayonnaise type, low-calorie	2 table-spoons[2]	30
Soft margarine[1]	1 teaspoon	5
Soybean lecithin	1 teaspoon	5
Monounsaturated Fat		
Avocado	1/8 (4-inch diameter)	25
Guacamole dip	2 table-spoons	25
Non-dairy creamer, liquid	2 table-spoons	30
Nuts[3]		
Almonds	7 whole, 1 tablespoon slivered	10
Brazil	2 whole	10
Cashews	5 medium	10
Chestnuts	2	15
Filberts, hazelnuts	5	10
Macadamia	4 whole	10
Peanuts		
Spanish	20 whole	10
Virginia	10 whole	10
Pecans	2 large	10
Pine nuts	¼ ounce	10
Pistachio	15	10
Walnuts	3 halves	10

Monounsaturated Fat	Serving Size	Grams
Nut butters	1 teaspoon	10
Nuts, chopped	1 table-spoon	10
Olives[3]	5 small	50
Olive oil	1 teaspoon	5
Peanut oil	1 teaspoon	5
Seeds	1 table-spoon	10
Pumpkin		
Sesame		
Sunflower		
Seed butters	1 teaspoon	10
Shortening	1 teaspoon	5
Stick margarine	1 teaspoon	5
Saturated Fat		
Bacon[3]	1 slice	10
Butter	1 teaspoon	5
Cocoa butter	1 teaspoon	5
Coconut oil	1 teaspoon	5
Coconut, shredded, unsweetened	1 table-spoon	10
Cream cheese	1 table-spoon	15
Cream		
Half-and-half	3 table-spoons	45
Light, sour	2 table-spoons	30
Whipped, unsweetened	2 table-spoons	15
Whipping, heavy	1 table-spoon	15
Lard	1 teaspoon	5
Non-dairy creamer, powdered	5 teaspoons	10
Palm oil	1 teaspoon	5
Pate de foie gras[3]	2 teaspoons	10
Salt pork[3]	¾-inch cube	15

---

[1]Made primarily with corn, cottonseed, safflower, soy or sunflower oil.
[2]Or see container for amount equivalent to 50 calories.
[3]May be high in sodium depending on manufacturer.

Fats are of both animal and vegetable origin. Animal fats are higher in saturated fat than most vegetable oils. It is not a good idea to use highly saturated fats exclusively. Oils are fats that remain liquid at room temperature and are usually of vegetable origin. Common fats obtained from vegetables are corn oil and peanut oil. Some of the common animal fats are butter and bacon. Since all fats are concentrated sources of calories, foods on this list should be measured carefully to control weight. To plan a diet low in saturated fat, select only those exchanges that are listed as polyunsaturated and monounsaturated fat.

P/S Ratio varies greatly in margarines. Read the label carefully. Most prepared foods must list ingredients in descending order of amount contained in the food. Select margarines made from vegetable oils only. The label is the key. The ingredient listed first is the major ingredient. A margarine that lists liquid vegetable oil as the first ingredient is low in saturated fat, high in polyunsaturated fat. For example, the ingredients may be listed as follows: liquid corn oil, partially hydrogenated corn oil (which means that liquid corn oil is the major ingredient), and so on.

P/S Ratio varies greatly in non-dairy creamers. Select non-dairy creamers that do not contain coconut oil. A non-dairy creamer that contains coconut oil is high in saturated fat and low in polyunsaturated fat. The powder non-dairy creamers (most of which contain coconut oil) are higher in saturated fat than the liquid non-dairy creamers.

I. FREE FOODS
(No Calories)

Another tip for using the exchange lists is to remember that there are certain foods you can use in unlimited amounts when planning your meals.

Beverages
Bouillon (without fat)[1]
Carbonated beverages, unsweetened or artificially sweetened
Coffee
Consomme (without fat)[1]
Diet drinks (read label for calorie content)
Mineral waters
Tea

Food

Celery
Chicory
Chinese cabbage
Cucumbers
Endive

Escarole
Gelatin, unsweetened or artificially sweetened
Lettuce
Pickles, unsweetened[1]
Watercress

Seasonings (No Salt)

Allspice
Almond extract
Anise seed
Basil
Bay leaf
Bouillon cube, low-sodium dietetic
Caraway seed
Cardamon
Cassia
Celery, leaves, seed
Chervil
Chili powder (no added salt)
Chives
Cilantro
Cinnamon
Cloves
Coriander
Cumin

Curry
Garlic, juice, powder
Ginger
Horseradish root, or prepared without salt
Juniper
Lemon juice or extract
Lime
Marjoram
Mace
Maple extract
Marjoram
Meat tenderizers, low-sodium dietetic
Mint
Mustard, dry or seed
Nutmeg
Onion, juice, powder
Orange extract

Oregano
Paprika
Parsley or flakes
Pepper, fresh green or red
Pepper, black, red or white
Peppermint extract
Pimento peppers
Poppyseed
Poultry seasoning
    (no added salt)
Pumpkin spice
Purslane
Rosemary
Saffron

Sage
Salt substitutes (if recom-
    mended by your physician)
Savory
Sorrel
Tarragon
Thyme
Turmeric
Vanilla extract
Vinegar
Walnut extract
Wine (in cooking), table

Seasonings (High Salt)
Baking powder, soda
Bouillon cube, regular
Celery salt
Chili sauce
Garlic salt
Horseradish, uncreamed,
    prepared with salt
Meat extracts
Meat tenderizers
Monosodium glutamate

Mustard, prepared
Onion salt
Pickles, unsweetened
Salt
Seasoning salts
Soy sauce
Tabasco sauce
Wine (in cooking),
    "Cooking Wine"
Worcestershire sauce

[1]Items are high in sodium.

J. ADDITIONAL LIST

If you wish to omit sweets from your diet, you may choose a serving of food from any of the exchange lists to supplement your entry calorie level. The Senate Select Committee on Nutrition and Human Needs recommends to increase fruit, vegetable and whole grains when increased calories are needed. For example, choose a serving representing 50 calories from vegetable list C or fruit list D. Accordingly, a serving representing 100 calories may come from the bread list E. However, if desserts or alcohol are desired, the foods below can be added to entry level calorie level to increase calories. The desserts, drinks, and sweets that we have listed contain approximately 100 calories per serving. Calorie levels are somewhat similar for the sugars and sweeteners listed below. They can be substituted, teaspoon for teaspoon. It is hard to tell how much sugar has been added to foods like peanut butter, catsup, or ready-to-eat cereal. Read the label. Ingredients are listed in order of predominance. If sugar or some other caloric sweetener[1] comes first, you know there is more sugar than anything else. It is a great deal easier to control the amount of sugar in your food, if you add it yourself.

Beverages	Serving Size	Grams
Alcoholic[2]		
Distilled liquors (80 proof)		
Liqueurs	1 ounce	30
Anisette (112 calories)	1 ounce	30
Apricot Brandy (98 calories)	1 ounce	30
Benedictine (105 calories)	1 ounce	30
Creme de menthe (100 calories)	1 ounce	30
Curacao (83 calories)	1 ounce	30
Brandy (105 calories)	1 ounce	30
Gin, dry (105 calories)	1½ ounces	45
Rum (105 calories)	1½ ounces	45
Vodka (105 calories)	1½ ounces	45
Whiskey, rye (119 calories)	1½ ounces	45
Whiskey, scotch (105 calories)	1½ ounces	45
Wines		
California, red (102 calories)	4 ounces	120
California, sauterne (102 calories)	4 ounces	120
Champagne, domestic, dry (100 calories)	5 ounces	150
Dubonet (96 calories)	3 ounces	90
French vermouth or madeira (95 calories)	3 ounces	90
Port or muscatel (95 calories)	2 ounces	60

Sake (100 calories)	2 ounces	60
Sherry, dry, domestic (85 calories)	2 ounces	60
Vermouth, Italian (100 calories)	2 ounces	60
Malt Liquors (American)		
Ale, mild (104 calories)	8 ounces	240
Beer (114 calories)	8 ounces	240
Mixed Drinks, cocktails (approximate from recipes)		
Daiquiri (112 calories)	3 ounces	90
Eggnog, Christmas type (82 calories)	1 ounce	30
Gin rickey (94 calories)	2½ ounces	75
High Ball (103 calories)	5 ounces	150
Manhattan (100 calories)	2 ounces	60
Martini (105 calories)	2½ ounce	75
Mint Julep (106 calories)	5 ounces	150
Old Fashioned (108 calories)	2 ounces	60
Planter's Punch (105 calories)	2 ounces	60
Rum Sour (99 calories)	2 ounces	60
Tom Collins (90 calories)	5 ounces	150
Carbonated, sweetened (7-Up, Coke, etc.)	8 ounces	240
Fruit punch	8 ounces	240
Hot chocolate	½ cup	120
Desserts[4]		
Apple Brown Betty	¼ cup	60
Brownie (1¾-inch × 1¾-inch × ⅞-inch)	1	20
Cakes[3]		
Chocolate (8-inch diameter × 3-inch high)		
no frosting	1-inch arch (1 ounce)	30
with frosting	¾-inch arch (1 ounce)	30
Fruitcake (1 pound loaf) (7-inch diameter × 2¼-inch high)	1 slice	30
Ginger bread (1½-inch × ½-inch × 2¼-inch cube)	1 ounce	30
Pound cake (8½-inch × 3½-inch × 3-inch loaf)	1 slice	20
Vanilla, yellow (8-inch diameter × 3-inch high)		
no frosting	1-inch arch	30
with frosting	¾-inch arch	30
Candy		
Hard	1 ounce	30
Chocolate	¾ ounce	20

Item	Serving Size	Grams
Nuts	¾ ounce	20
Cookies[3]	2 small (2-inch diameter)	20
Cranberry sauce	3 table-spoons	70
Cupcakes[3]		
no frosting	1 (2½-inch diameter)	30
with frosting	1 (2¼-inch diameter)	30
Custard	⅓ cup	90
Doughnut, cake and yeast (3½ inch diameter × 1-inch high)	1 (⅞ ounce)	25
Fudge	1 cubic inch	20
Gelatin, sweetened	⅔ cup	160
Ice Cream	⅓ cup	50
Ice Milk	½ cup	65
Pie[3] (9-inch diameter)	1-inch arch 1/22 of pie)	33
Pudding	⅓ cup	80
Semi-sweet chocolate	¾ ounce	20
Sherbet	⅓ cup	60
Tapioca		
Fruit	⅓ cup	80
Cream pudding	½ cup	80
Sugars		
Brown sugar, corn syrup, honey, jam, jelly, maple syrup, marmalade, molasses, white sugar	2 table-spoons	40
Miscellaneous		
Cocoa, dry powder	1 ounce	28
Malt, dry	1 ounce	28

---

[1]Words used on labels to describe sugar and caloric sweeteners include sugar, sucrose, dextrose, fructose, corn syrup, corn sweeteners, natural sweeteners, honey, invert sugar.

[2]We are not advocating the use of alcoholic beverages, but are indicating where they fit if you choose to use them.

[3]The weights, measures and caloric values are considered reasonable estimates, but they should be used realizing that specific samples will vary.

[4]Most pre-packaged or prepared desserts are high in sodium.

Recipes

APPLE AND ENDIVE SALAD

2 tablespoons lemon juice
4 small apples, cored into ¼ inch slices
½ cup celery, diced
4 small endives, cored, cut into 2-inch strips*
2 tablespoons oil
12 whole broken walnuts
1 tablespoon minced mint or parsley leaves
Drizzle lemon juice over sliced apples; toss well. Mix in celery, endives, and oil. Just before serving, stir in walnuts. Garnish with mint or parsley. Serves 4. Time: 15 minutes.
Each serving = 180 calories
    1 Vegetable Exchange (B)
    1 Fruit Exchange (D)
    3 Fat Exchanges (H)
*If not available, 2 cups torn lettuce may be substituted.

APRICOT-ALMOND TAPIOCA

1 can (16-ounce) sliced apricots* (packed in natural juice, no
   sugar added)
½ cup wheat germ
6 tablespoons slivered almonds
2 tablespoons quick-cooking tapioca
1 tablespoon honey
2 teaspoons lemon juice
1 teaspoon rum extract
2 teaspoons unsalted margarine (corn oil)
Drain liquid from apricots reserving 1¼ cup liquid. Arrange apricot slices in shallow 1½ quart baking dish. Sprinkle with wheat germ and almonds. Combine tapioca, honey, lemon juice, rum extract and reserved apricot juice. Cook over medium heat, stirring constantly, until thickened. Stir in margarine until melted. Pour over fruit mixture. Bake at 375°F for 15 minutes. Serve warm. Serves 8. Time: 40 minutes.
Each serving = 126 calories
    1 Fruit Exchange (D)
    ½ Bread Exchange (E)
    1 Fat Exchange (H)
*Peaches may be used as substitution

BAKED HALIBUT

1 pound halibut steak (boneless)
¼ teaspoon paprika
Pinch of cayenne
Juice of 1 lemon
¼ cup chopped onion
4 teaspoons margarine (corn oil)
¼ cup dry white wine
Thin green pepper strips

Sprinkle fish with seasonings and lemon juice. Marinate covered in refrigerator for 1 hour, turning once. Saute onion in margarine. Place steaks in baking dish. Sprinkle with wine and spread with sauteed onion. Top with green pepper strips. Bake in hot oven (400 to 425°F) for 10 minutes. Serves 4. Time: 25 minutes.
Each serving = 210 calories
  1 Vegetable Exchange (B)
  3 Animal Protein Exchanges (F1)
  1 Fat Exchange (H)

BANANA MILKSHAKE

1 cup non-fat milk or buttermilk
1 banana (or may substitute any 2 servings of fruit)
Vanilla extract (to taste)

Combine ingredients in blender. May use frozen fruit (no sugar added) for a cold frosted drink. Banana may be peeled and frozen, too. Serves 1. Time: 20 seconds.
Each serving = 160 calories
  1 Milk Exchange (A1)
  2 Fruit Exchanges (D)

BEAN AND BEEF ENCHILADAS

4 large corn or flour tortillas (6-inch diameter)
2 teaspoons oil
½ green pepper, chopped
¼ cup onions, chopped
1½ tablespoons chili powder
1 clove garlic, crushed
½ teaspoon onion powder
1½ cups cooked kidney beans
2 ounces lean ground beef (less than 10% fat)
12 ounces pureed tomatoes
2 ounces grated skim milk cheese

Cook onion and green pepper in oil until soft. In separate pan, sauté beef until cooked; drain excess fat. Drain beans and mash. Add 1 tablespoon of the chili powder, the garlic, 2 tablespoons of the tomato puree, and the mashed beans and beef to the onions and green pepper. Mix well. Place ¼ of the bean and beef mixture on each tortilla. Roll tortillas* and place in a baking dish. In a bowl combine remainder of tomato puree and the rest of the spices. Pour the tomato puree sauce over the enchiladas, and top each with ¼ of the grated cheese. Cover and bake at 350°F for 20 minutes, until cheese on top is melted. Serves 2. Two tortillas each. Time: 50 minutes.

Each serving = 490 calories
  2 Vegetable Exchanges (B)
  2 Bread Exchanges (E)
  2 Animal Protein Exchanges (F1)
  1 Vegetable Protein Exchange (G1)
  1 Fat Exchange (H)

*If tortillas are hard to roll, they may be softened by steaming. Place 2 tortillas at a time in a strainer and place them over, *not in,* boiling water. Cover and steam 2 to 3 minutes until softened.

Variations: Red pepper, cayenne pepper, or tabasco sauce may be added to filling and/or sauce.

BEAN AND CARROT VINAIGRETTE

  3 cups cooked dry, small white beans, drained (or 3 8-ounce
    cans, drained)
  2 cups carrots, cooked, sliced
  ⅓ cup chopped green pepper
  ½ cup thinly sliced purple onion
  2½ tablespoons chopped parsley
  2 tablespoons vinegar
  8 teaspoons oil
  ½ teaspoon dijon-style mustard
  Dash of pepper

Place vegetables in shallow bowl. Combine vinegar, oil, mustard and pepper; pour over vegetables and refrigerate overnight. Serves 4. Time: 20 minutes.

Each serving = 280 calories
  1 Vegetable Exchange (B)
  1 Vegetable Exchange (C)
  1 Vegetable Protein Exchange (G1)
  2 Fat Exchanges (H)

BEAN BURRITO

3 cups cooked kidney beans
¼ cup water or stock
½ cup onions chopped
2 medium tomatoes, chopped (or ⅔ cup canned)
1 clove garlic, minced
1 teaspoon chili powder
Pinch cayenne
4 tortillas (flour or corn) (6-inch)

Cook beans with onion, garlic, chili, cayenne, water or stock, and tomatoes over medium heat until beans are soft (20 minutes). Mash bean mixture with potato masher until smooth or use food processor. Place ¼ of hot bean mixture in tortilla.

Optional: Green onions, diced cucumber and tomatoes, or shredded lettuce may be added on top of bean mixture in burrito.

Note: To warm tortilla, sprinkle with water and warm in 350°F oven for 10 minutes, or microwave for 30 seconds. Serves 4. Time: 20 minutes.

Each serving = 250 calories
   1 Vegetable Exchange (B)
   1 Bread Exchange (E)
   1 Vegetable Protein Exchange (G1)

BROCCOLI A L'ORANGE

1½ pounds broccoli, separated into spears
Water
2 tablespoons margarine (corn oil)
2 teaspoons flour
½-1 teaspoon grated orange peel
½ cup orange juice (unsweetened)
Dash of ground nutmeg

Steam broccoli in small amount of boiling water (covered) until tender. Drain. In a sauce pan melt margarine. Stir in flour and orange peel. Gradually stir in orange juice and nutmeg. Cook over medium heat until thickened 3-4 minutes. Serve over broccoli. Serves 6. Time: 20 minutes.

Each serving = 70 calories
   1 Vegetable Exchange (B)
   1 Fat Exchange (H)

CABBAGE AND APPLE SLAW

1 tablespoon minced onion
½ teaspoon caraway seed
½ teaspoon dry mustard
¼ teaspoon white pepper
3 tablespoons white vinegar
4 teaspoons sugar
4 teaspoons margarine
4 cups finely shredded cabbage
1 cup unpeeled, diced apple

Combine onion, caraway seed, dry mustard, pepper, vinegar and sugar. Blend thoroughly. Set aside. In a large skillet melt margarine. Add cabbage and apple and sauté over medium heat for 3 minutes. Stir in vinegar mixture and simmer on low heat, stirring occasionally, until apples and cabbage are tender, about 5 minutes. Serves 4. Time: 20 minutes.

Each serving = 110 calories
    1 Vegetable Exchange (B)
    1 Fruit Exchange (D)
    1 Fat Exchange (H)

CHICKEN AND HAZELNUT SALAD

¼ cup plain low-fat yogurt
6 tablespoons mayonnaise
¼ teaspoon curry powder
1 tablespoon skim milk
2½ cups diced, cooked, white chicken meat (12 ounces)
1 cup celery, sliced
2 tablespoons chopped onion
6 ounces chopped hazelnuts*
Lettuce leaves

Mix together yogurt, mayonnaise, curry powder and milk. Add chicken, celery and onion. Toss well. Chill thoroughly. Just before serving, mix in hazelnuts. Serve on lettuce leaves. Serves 6. Time: 40 minutes.

Each serving = 420 calories
    2 Animal Protein Exchanges (F1)
    1 Vegetable Protein Exchange (G3)
    3 Fat Exchanges (H)
*Slivered almonds may be substituted if hazelnuts are unavailable.

CHICKEN PILAU

4 teaspoons oil (corn)
1 cup bulgar wheat or rice
2 tablespoons finely chopped onion
2½ cups chicken broth
1 teaspoon oregano
1½ cups chopped chicken, cooked (about 12 ounces)
2 tablespoons minced parsley
¼ teaspoon pepper
Paprika

Warm oil in heavy skillet; add bulgar and onion. Stir and cook until golden brown. Pour broth and seasonings over bulgar; cover, bring to boil. Reduce heat, simmer 10 minutes. Add chicken, simmer 5 minutes more. Sprinkle with paprika. Serves 4. Time: 45 minutes. Each serving = 350 calories

2 Bread Exchanges (E)
3 Animal Protein Exchanges (F1)
1 Fat Exchange (H)

CHINESE BEEF WITH VEGETABLES

1 pound flank steak
1 tablespoon soy sauce
½ cup water or beef broth or stock
¾ cup broccoli flowers
½ cup fresh mushrooms, sliced
¼ cup celery, sliced
1 cube beef bouillon (eliminate if broth or stock is used)
½ cup bean sprouts
¼ cup Chinese greens (bok choy, cabbage or other leafy greens)
1 pound firm tofu, cubed
1 tablespoon cornstarch in 2 tablespoons water
1 medium tomato, cut in wedges
1 ounce Spanish peanuts (about 40 whole peanuts, unsalted)

Score steak, marinade in soy sauce and ¼ cup water or broth 10 minutes, turning once. Reserve marinade. Broil steak on rack for 6 minutes; turn and broil an additional 4 minutes (will be rare). Cool, cut into thick slices. Set aside. In a skillet combine ¼ cup water or broth, broccoli, mushrooms, celery and broth mix. Cook over high heat 2 minutes, stirring occasionally. Add reserved marinade, mix well. When vegetables are tender yet crisp, add steak slices, bean

sprouts, greens and tofu. Stir, then add cornstarch, stirring until mixture thickens. Add tomato wedges, and peanuts; mix well. Serves 4. Time: 35 minutes.
Each serving = 320 calories
  1 Vegetable Exchange (B)
  3 Animal Protein Exchanges (F1)
  1 Vegetable Protein Exchange (G2)
  1 Fat Exchange (H)

COQ AU VIN

  6 4-ounce chicken breasts, deboned, skin removed
  ¼ cup flour in a paper bag with freshly ground pepper
  2 tablespoons margarine
  1 cup chicken stock
  ½ cup burgundy
  1 teaspoon thyme
  1 teaspoon marjoram
  2 tablespoons chopped parsley
  2 small white boiling onions, peeled
  4 celery stalks, whole

Put chicken in bag of flour and shake until well coated. Brown the chicken in margarine. Heat the stock and add to the pan. Add wine, herbs and onions. Cover with celery. Cook slowly for 1 hour over low heat. Discard celery and remove chicken and onions to a serving dish. Simmer gravy until reduced slightly. Spoon sauce over chicken and onions. Serves 6. Time: 1½ hours.
Each serving = 235 calories
  1 Vegetable Exchange (B)
  3 Animal Protein Exchanges (F1)
  1 Fat Exchange (H)

COQUILLES SAINT-JACQUES

  1 pound scallops
  ¼ cup dry white wine
  ½ pound mushrooms, sliced
  1 bay leaf
Sauce:
  4 teaspoons margarine (corn oil)
  4 teaspoons flour
  1 cup evaporated low-fat milk
  1 tablespoon chopped parsley
  ¼ teaspoon freshly ground black pepper
  2 tablespoons sherry
  Paprika

Combine scallops with wine, mushrooms, and bay leaf in skillet. Bring to boil, reduce heat and simmer, covered, 2 minutes. Remove from heat. Melt margarine in sauce pan. Blend in flour until smooth. Add milk all at once. Cook and stir until thick and bubbly. Add parsley, pepper and stir in sherry. Stir scallop mixture into sauce. Put into shallow baking dish. Cover pan with foil and bake at 375°F for 15 minutes. Uncover and bake 5 minutes longer or until sauce bubbles. Remove from oven and sprinkle with paprika. Serves 4. Time: 30 minutes.

Each serving = 270 calories
   ½ Milk Exchange (A2)
   3 Animal Protein Exchanges (F1)
   1 Fat Exchange (H)

Variations: Cod, sole fillet, or any boneless, firm white fish may be substituted for scallops.

CREAMY CUCUMBER SOUP

   1 medium cucumber, peeled, seeded, diced (1 cup)
   2 tablespoons green onion, chopped
   3 teaspoons margarine (corn oil)
   2 teaspoons cornstarch
   ¾ cup stock (chicken)
   ½ cup low-fat milk
   ¼ teaspoon dried dill weed (or 1 teaspoon fresh)
   ¼ teaspoon grated lemon rind
   Dash pepper, ground
   ½ cup low-fat plain yogurt
   Dash of garlic powder (optional)

Cook cucumber and onion in margarine about 5 minutes in a sauce-pan. Stir in cornstarch. Add stock, milk, dill, lemon and pepper; mix well. Cook over low to medium heat, stirring frequently, until thickened (about 10 minutes). Puree mixture in a blender until smooth. Stir cucumber mixture into yogurt. Pour into covered container and chill. Garnish with mint leaf. Serves 4. Time: 20 minutes.

Each ¾ cup serving = 70 calories
   1 Vegetable Exchange (B)
   1 Fat Exchange (H)

CREPE

   1 cup unbleached flour
   1½ cups non-fat milk
   1 egg, beaten
   2 teaspoons oil (corn)

Combine flour, milk and egg; beat until blended. Chill batter. Lightly grease a 6-inch nonstick pan with some of the oil. Place pan over medium heat until pan is hot. Remove pan from heat and spoon in 2 tablespoons of the batter. Tilt the pan until the batter is spread evenly over the bottom. Crepe should slide easily from pan when cooked. Repeat, greasing skillet as needed. Yield: 18 crepes. Time: 30 minutes.

Each serving = 35 calories
½ Bread Exchange (E)

CURRIED CHICKEN

1 pound chicken breasts, boned
4 teaspoons vegetable oil (corn oil)
½ pound sliced mushrooms
¼ cup chopped onion
1 tablespoon curry powder
¼ cup chopped parsley
1 chicken bouillon cube in 1 cup boiling water (or use 1 cup chicken broth or stock)
1 teaspoon arrowroot powder or cornstarch
Tumeric to taste

Skin chicken breasts and cut into 1-inch pieces. Sauté chicken, mushrooms, and onions in oil until lightly browned on all sides. Stir in curry powder and parsley. Dissolve bouillon cube in boiling water; add to chicken mixture. Stir in arrowroot. Simmer for 20 minutes, until chicken is cooked, stirring often, as curry burns easily. Add a pinch of tumeric. Serves 4. Time: 45 minutes.

Each serving = 220 calories
1 Vegetable Exchange (B)
3 Animal Protein Exchanges (F1)
1 Fat Exchange (H)

FISH CHOWDER

1 cup uncooked potato cubes
1 cup sliced carrots
1 cup coarsely chopped onion
⅓ cup celery, sliced
8 peppercorns
1 bay leaf
Cold water (or broth)
12 ounces fillet of cod (boneless)
¼ cup margarine (corn oil)
¼ cup white flour
4 cups low-fat milk
4 tablespoons chopped parsley

Heat potatoes, carrots, onion, celery, peppercorns and bay leaf in cold water or broth (to cover) in a large sauce pan to a boil. Reduce heat and simmer 15 minutes. Add fish and simmer another 15 minutes or until fish flakes easily with a fork. Remove fish, vegetables and seasonings. Boil broth until reduced to 1 cup. Discard peppercorns and bay leaf. Break fish into chunks. Melt margarine. Blend in flour. Stir in milk and reduced broth. Cook over medium heat, stirring constantly until mixture comes to a boil. Add fish and vegetables. Heat through. Serve hot garnished with parsley. Serves 4. Time: 45 minutes.

Each 2-cup serving = 475 calories
  1 Milk Exchange (A2)
  1 Vegetable Exchange (C)
  1 Bread Exchange (E)
  2 Animal Protein Exchanges (F1)
  3 Fat Exchanges (H)

FRUIT CREPES

Apricot
  1 teaspoon margarine (corn oil)
  6 apricots, thinly sliced
  1 cup unsweetened apricot nectar
Peach
  1 teaspoon margarine (corn oil)
  3 medium peaches, thinly sliced
  1 cup unsweetened peach nectar
Strawberry
  1 teaspoon margarine (corn oil)
  3 cups strawberries
  1 cup unsweetened apple juice

  2 tablespoons Cointreau or other orange liqueur
  1 tablespoon cornstarch
  ¼ teaspoon vanilla extract
  2 teaspoons water
  6 Crepes — see recipe
  ¾ ounce chopped almonds

Melt margarine in skillet. Add fruit, juice, liqueur and mix. Cover and cook over low heat until fruit is soft, about 10 minutes. Mix cornstarch with vanilla and water. Stir into fruit mixture, stir until thickens. Fill each crepe with ¼ cup fruit. Roll and top with remaining sauce. Top with ¾ ounce chopped almonds. Serves 6. Time: 30 minutes.

Each serving = 120 calories
  1 Fruit Exchange (D)
  ½ Bread Exchange (E)
  1 Fat Exchange (H)

GRAPE AND HAM SALAD

48 grapes (green, red or blue/black), halved
8 ounces cooked ham strips
2 cups shredded head lettuce
2 cups torn leaf lettuce
½ cup thinly sliced onion
Vinaigrette dressing*
Combine all ingredients; toss lightly. Serves 4. Time: 10 minutes.
Each serving = 210 calories
   1 Vegetable Exchange (B)
   1 Fruit Exchange (D)
   2 Animal Protein Exchanges (F1)
   1 Fat Exchange (H)
*Vinaigrette dressing: Combine 4 teaspoons oil, 2 tablespoons vinegar, 2 teaspoons horseradish, ½ teaspoon Worcestershire sauce, ⅛ teaspoon pepper, and dash cayenne.

KAHLUA PEARS MERINGUE

1¼ cups white wine
¼ cup Kahlua
1 tablespoon lemon juice
4 tablespoons honey
6 pears, (2½-inch diameter; 3½-inch high) about 2½
   pounds
2 tablespoons Anisette liqueur or Brandy
3 egg whites
¼ teaspoon cream of tarter
1. Bring wine, Kahlua, lemon juice and 2 tablespoons of the honey to simmer over medium heat. Pare, quarter, and core pears, dropping them into simmering liquid as they are ready. Simmer pears, covered, 20 to 30 minutes, until just tender, depending on ripeness of pears. Add Anisette liqueur. Remove pan from heat. Place pears, cavity down, in a shallow 9-inch pie or quiche plate. Pour poaching liquid over them.
2. In a bowl, beat egg whites and cream of tartar until foamy; add 2 tablespoons of honey; whip until stiff peaks form.
3. Pile meringue in a ring around pie or quiche plate. Bake in preheated, 375-degree oven until meringue is golden in color, about 10 minutes. Serve immediately. Serves 6. Time: 45 minutes.
Each serving = 160 calories
   4 Fruit Exchanges (D)

LAMB AND VEGETABLES WITH LIME

Part I:
  2 tablespoons soy sauce
  ¼ cup lime juice
  ½ cup stock (chicken or beef) or consomme
  Ground pepper to season
  ½ teaspoon ground coriander
  2 cloves garlic, crushed
  2 scallions, chopped
  1 pound lean lamb cut into 1½-inch cubes (trim all visible fat)
Part II:
  ½ pound fresh mushrooms
  ½ pound cherry tomatoes
  ¼ pound green peppers
  ¼ pound cauliflower
  ½ pound small boiling onions

Combine Part I for marinade. Stir to coat. Refrigerate covered several hours or overnight. Alternate meat cubes and vegetables on skewers. Place on broiler rack. Brush with marinade mixture. Broil about 4 inches from heat, turning occasionally until meat and vegetables are tender, about 12 to 15 minutes. Serves 4. Time: 25 minutes.

Each serving = 215 calories
  1 Vegetable Exchange (B)
  1 Vegetable Exchange (C)
  3 Animal Protein Exchanges (F1)

LEMON-PINEAPPLE CHEESE PIE

  1½ cups graham cracker crumbs
  8 teaspoons margarine, melted (corn oil)
  3-ounce package lemon-flavored gelatin
  1 cup boiling water
  1½ pounds low-fat cottage cheese (put through a sieve)
  2 tablespoons sugar
  1 teaspoon grated lemon peel
  8½ ounce can crushed pineapple, packed in own juice
  1 tablespoon water
  2 teaspoons cornstarch

Mix crumbs and margarine, press into bottom of a 9-inch pie pan. Bake at 350°F for 10 minutes. Cool. Dissolve gelatin in boiling water and cool until lukewarm. Blend cottage cheese, sugar and lemon peel with hand mixer. Slowly add dissolved gelatin and mix well. Pour into crust and chill until firm. Stir cornstarch and water in a sauce pan until smooth. Blend pineapple and its juice into corn-starch mixture and bring to a boil, stirring constantly. Cool 15 minutes, spread over cake, and chill 1 hour or more. Serves 8. Time: 30 minutes.

Each serving = 280 calories
- 1 Fruit Exchange (D)
- 1 Bread Exchange (E)
- 2 Animal Protein Exchanges (F1)
- 1 Fat Exchange (H)

LEMON POTATOES WITH DILL

6 small baking potatoes
⅓ cup chopped onion
1 clove garlic, minced
2 tablespoons margarine (corn oil)
½ cup hot skim milk
2 teaspoons grated lemon peel
¼ teaspoon white pepper
1 tablespoon chopped fresh dill weed, or 1 teaspoon dried
1 tablespoon finely chopped parsley or chervil
Paprika

Bake potatoes (about 40 to 45 minutes at 400°F). Cool enough to handle. Meanwhile, sauté onion and garlic in margarine until tender. Scoop out potatoes, being careful to keep skins from breaking. Mash potato. Beat in sauteed onion mixture, hot milk, lemon peel, and pepper. Mix in dill and parsley. Pile mashed potato mixture in skins. Sprinkle with paprika. Bake at 400°F about 30 minutes, or until lightly browned. Serves 6. Time: 1 hour 40 minutes.

Each serving = 120 calories
- 1 Bread Exchange (E)
- 1 Fat Exchange (H)

LEMON SOLE

¼ cup chopped onion
2 cups sliced, fresh mushrooms
2 tablespoons margarine (corn oil)
1½ pounds sole fillet
¼ cup dry white wine
2 tablespoons lemon juice
1 tablespoon chopped parsley
1 teaspoon oregano
⅛ teaspoon pepper

Sauté onions and mushrooms in margarine until tender in a large

skillet. Lay sole in pan and sprinkle remaining ingredients over fish. Cover and simmer gently for 10 minutes. Serves 6. Time: 20 minutes.
Each serving = 220 calories
   1 Vegetable Exchange (B)
   3 Animal Protein Exchanges (F1)
   1 Fat Exchange (H)

LIMA BEAN CASSEROLE

1 jar (4-ounce) whole pimentos
3 cups large, dry, lima beans, cooked
1 cup finely chopped onions
3 cloves garlic, crushed
4 teaspoons margarine (corn oil)
2 teaspoons red pepper flakes
1½ tablespoons lemon juice
Dash white pepper
2 tablespoons minced parsley
¼ cup chopped celery

Whirl pimentos in blender until smooth. Drain lima beans, reserving ¼ cup liquid. Saute onions and garlic in margarine over low heat 10 minutes. Stir in pimentos, beans, liquid, spices, parsley and celery. Pour into 1 quart casserole. Bake at 350°F, covered, about 35 minutes. Serves 4. Time: 45 minutes.
Each serving = 220 calories
   1 Vegetable Exchange (B)
   1 Vegetable Protein Exchange (G1)
   1 Fat Exchange (H)

LOW-CALORIE DRESSING[1]

French Dressing

1 cup tomato juice
2 tablespoons lemon juice
½ teaspoon dried oregano
Pinch of garlic powder
Pinch of pepper

Makes 1 cup, with 7 calories per 2 tablespoons. Time: 5 minutes.

[1]Commercially prepared low-calorie dressings may be substituted for those in our menus. Check calories on label for comparison and adjust quantities accordingly.

Mustard Vinaigrette Dressing

2 tablespoons vinegar
¾ cup water
1 clove garlic, whole
2 teaspoons oil
2 teaspoons dijon mustard
Dash pepper

Allow garlic to stand in mixture overnight; then remove. Makes 1 cup, with 12 calories per 2 tablespoons. Time: 5 minutes.

Russian Dressing

1 cup low-fat cottage cheese
½ cup tomato juice
¼ cup lemon juice or vinegar
1 teaspoon dijon mustard
⅛ teaspoon pepper, ground
Dash of chili powder

Combine in blender or food processor until smooth. Makes 2 cups, with 14 calories per 2 tablespoons. Time: 5 minutes.

Creamy Herb Dressing

1 cup low-fat yogurt
½ cup evaporated non-fat milk
2 cloves garlic, chopped
1 teaspoon dried basil
1 teaspoon dried dill or tarragon
1 teaspoon dried sage
1 teaspoon dried chervil
¼ teaspoon white pepper, ground

Combine in blender or food processor until smooth. Makes 1½ cups, with 14 calories per 2 tablespoons. Time: 5 minutes.

Note: Fresh herbs (1 tablespoon) if available may be substituted for dried herbs (1 teaspoon) in all recipes.

MOLDED FRUIT SALAD

1 tablespoon unflavored gelatin
2 cups unsweetened fruit, juice (do not use pineapple juice; it
    will not gel)
1 cup sliced fruit, such as peaches, pears, apples, bananas, berries

Mix together ¼ cup juice and gelatin in a bowl. Measure another ¼ cup juice, boil it, then add hot juice to the preceding mixture and stir until gelatin is dissolved. Add remaining juice and stir. Refrigerate to set. After the gelatin begins to set a little, add the sliced fruit and put gelatin into an 8-inch ring-mold. Return gelatin to refrigerator until firm. Turn out onto lettuce bed on large plate. Serves 8; about ⅓ cup each. Time: 30 minutes.
Each serving = 48 calories
  1 Fruit Exchange (D)

MUSHROOM-RICE SALAD WITH PINE NUTS

  3 cups sliced mushrooms
  ½ cup chopped onion
  3 cloves garlic, crushed
  3 tablespoons chopped parsley
  2 teaspoons basil leaves, crushed (or 2 tablespoons fresh if
    available)
  ¼ teaspoon pepper
  3 teaspoons margarine (corn oil)
  2 cups cooked white rice
  3 tablespoons oil
  4 ounces pine nuts

Sauté mushrooms, onion, garlic, parsley, basil and pepper in margarine about 10 minutes, stirring frequently, until tender. Combine with rice, and oil. Chill. Add pine nuts before serving. Serves 4. Time: 25 minutes.
Each serving = 380 calories
  1 Vegetable Exchange (B)
  1 Vegetable Protein Exchange (G3)
  1 Bread Exchange (E)
  3 Fat Exchanges (H)

OATMEAL COOKIES

  ½ cup margarine, softened (corn oil)
  ½ cup firmly packed brown sugar
  1¼ cups unsifted whole wheat flour
  1 cup old-fashioned oats, uncooked
  ½ cup chopped English walnuts or pecans
  ⅓ cup seedless raisins
  1½ teaspoons ground cinnamon
  ½ teaspoon vanilla extract
  ¼ cup skim milk

Cream margarine with brown sugar. Stir in remaining ingredients. Form into balls using 1 tablespoon dough for each ball. Place on

ungreased baking sheet. Flatten with lightly floured bottom of a glass. Bake at 350°F about 15 minutes, or until done. Remove and put on wire rack. Yield: 2½ dozen. Time: 45 minutes.
Each cookie = 100 calories
    ½ Fruit Exchange (D)
    ½ Bread Exchange (E)
    1 Fat Exchange (H)

ORANGE CHEESE SOUFFLE

    3 eggs (separate yolks and whites)
    1¼ cups low-fat cottage cheese (uncreamed)
    1 teaspoon grated onion
    ½ cup orange juice
    ½ teaspoon dry mustard
    ¼ teaspoon tarragon
    ⅛ teaspoon pepper
    ½ teaspoon grated orange peel
    ¼ teaspoon cream of tartar

Mix all ingredients except egg whites and cream of tartar. In medium bowl, beat egg whites and cream of tartar until stiff but not dry. Fold egg white into egg yolk mixture. Spoon into four-quart casserole or souffle dish. Bake at 350°F for 30 to 40 minutes or until top is puffed and slightly brown. Serves 4. Time: 45 minutes.
Each serving = 130 calories
    2 Animal Protein Exchanges (F1,2)

PASTA ALLA PIEMONTESE

    1 pound lean ground beef (less than 10% fat)
    1½ cups sliced mushrooms
    ½ cup chopped onion
    2 large cloves garlic, crushed
    4 teaspoons oil (corn)
    2 pounds fresh tomatoes, peeled, cored and chopped (or 28 ounces canned tomatoes and liquid)
    2 cans (8 ounces each) tomato sauce
    ½ cup water (omit if canned tomatoes are used)
    ¼ teaspoon pepper
    1 teaspoon rosemary leaves
    8 ounces uncooked dry pasta (shells, fettucini, spaghetti, tagliarini) or 1 pound fresh pasta (amount should equal 4 cups cooked)

Brown meat thoroughly. Drain excess fat. Remove from pan. Sauté mushrooms, onion, and garlic in oil. Stir in tomatoes, tomato sauce, water, pepper and rosemary. Simmer uncovered for 20 minutes. Cover; reduce heat and continue cooking for 40 minutes. Add meat. Cover and simmer an additional 20 minutes.

Meanwhile, cook pasta according to package directions. Pour sauce over hot pasta and mix thoroughly. Serve at once. Serves 4. Time: 1½ hours.

Each serving = 500 calories
  2 Vegetable Exchanges (C)
  2 Bread Exchanges (E)
  3 Animal Protein Exchanges (F1)
  1 Fat Exchange (H)

PEA AND TURNIP BISQUE

3 cups stock (beef, chicken or vegetable)
1 pound turnips, peeled, quartered
1 large onion, quartered
2 cups frozen green peas (thawed)
8 teaspoons margarine (corn oil)
1 cup instant non-fat dry milk
⅛ teaspoon ground pepper
Dash nutmeg, ground

In a pressure cooker,* boil turnips and onions in stock until soft (about 5 minutes). Strain vegetables, reserving the stock. Blend vegetables with remaining ingredients in a blender until smooth and creamy, adding enough stock to moisten. Return pureed mixture to pot with remaining stock. Mix well and heat through, about 5 minutes. Serve topped with ground nutmeg. Serves 4. Time: 30 minutes.

Each 1½ cup serving = 270 calories
  1 Milk Exchange (A1)
  2 Vegetable Exchanges (C) (calories and nutrients similar to 1 Bread Exchange)
  2 Fat Exchanges (H)

*If pressure cooker is not used, vegetables may be chopped and cooked a little longer until soft.

RAGOUT OF BEEF WITH MARJORAM

1 pound boneless beef cut into 1-inch cubes
½ cup tomato juice
2 teaspoons Worcestershire sauce
1 teaspoon dried marjoram
¼ teaspoon pepper
½ cup onion, chopped
1 cup carrots, thinly sliced
2 cups diced potatoes
2 cups zucchini, thickly sliced
2 medium tomatoes, peeled, quartered

Combine all vegetables except zucchini and tomatoes in a skillet with seasonings and tomato juice. Simmer covered over low heat for

20 minutes. Meanwhile, broil meat on rack in oven until brown and cooked on all sides. Drain thoroughly on paper towel. Add zucchini, tomatoes and meat to skillet. Continue cooking 15 minutes (covered). Serves 4. Time: 50 minutes.

Each serving = 310 calories

   2 Vegetable Exchanges (C)

   1 Bread Exchange (E)

   3 Animal Protein Exchanges (F1)

RASBERRY-HONEY MUFFINS

1¾ cups whole wheat flour

2 teaspoons baking powder

1 teaspoon cinnamon

¼ teaspoon nutmeg

1 cup buttermilk

1 egg

⅓ cup safflower oil

¼ cup honey

½ cup chopped walnuts

1 cup raspberries* (fresh or frozen, drained)

Beat together buttermilk, egg, oil and honey. Combine flour, baking powder, cinnamon and nutmeg in a separate bowl and add to buttermilk mixture. Stir in walnuts and raspberries. Blend well. Bake in muffin cups at 400°F for 25 to 30 minutes. Makes 12 muffins. Time: 35 minutes.

Each serving = 200 calories

   1 Fruit Exchange (D)

   1 Bread Exchange (E)

   2 Fat Exchanges (H)

*Apricots, berries (all kinds) or peaches may be substituted.

RICE WITH CHILI

1 large onion, chopped

2 small scallions, chopped

1 clove garlic, minced

4 teaspoons margarine (corn oil)

½ green pepper, chopped

1 8-ounce can tomato sauce

1 whole, fresh tomato, chopped

3 cups kidney beans, cooked, drained

¼ teaspoon cumin powder

¼ teaspoon red pepper flakes

½ to ¾ teaspoon chili powder

2 tablespoons chopped parsley

½ cup water

2 cups cooked brown rice

Sauté onions, scallions and garlic in margarine. Add tomato sauce, water, tomato and green pepper; simmer for 30 minutes. Add kidney beans, spices and parsley to mixture. Cook over slow heat, covered, for 2 hours. Serve over brown rice. Serves 4. Time: 2½ hours.

Each serving = 320 calories
  1 Vegetable Exchange (C)
  1 Bread Exchange (E)
  1 Vegetable Protein Exchange (G1)
  1 Fat Exchange (H)

TOFU QUICHE

¼ cup onion chopped
1 cup chopped broccoli or spinach
8 large mushrooms, sliced
2 cloves garlic
¼ teaspoon pepper
¼ teaspoon curry powder
½ cup low-fat cottage cheese
8 ounces tofu
2 eggs
¼ teaspoon dry mustard
Dust pan with:
  1) 6 tablespoons wheat germ, or
  2) 4 (2¼-inch-square) graham cracker crumbs or
  3) 5 tablespoons whole wheat flour

Chop vegetables, sauté with spices in 2 teaspoons oil until partially cooked. Drain excess water.* Blend cottage cheese, tofu, eggs and mustard in food processor or blender. Add vegetables to cheese and tofu mixture. Pour mixture into dusted pie pan. Bake at 350°F for 30 minutes until center is firm. Serves 2. Time: 45 minutes.

Each serving = 350 calories
  1 Vegetable Exchange (B)
  1 Bread Exchange (E)
  2 Animal Protein Exchanges (F1,2)
  1 Vegetable Protein Exchange (G2)
  1 Fat Exchange (H)

*If frozen vegetables are used, be sure that they are thoroughly thawed and well drained before sauteeing, otherwise quiche will be watery.

TUNA-BEAN SALAD

3 cups dry, medium-size white beans, cooked, drained
⅓ cup chopped onion
4 tablespoons oil (corn)
8-ounces canned tuna (water-packed)
2 tablespoons wine vinegar
3 tablespoons chopped parsley
¼ teaspoon pepper
Combine all ingredients in a 2-quart bowl. Chill several hours.
Serves 4. Time: 15 minutes.
Each serving = 410 calories
   2 Animal Protein Exchanges (F1)
   1 Vegetable Protein Exchange (G1)
   3 Fat Exchanges (H)

PLAY PLANS FOR VARIOUS
CALORIE EXPENDITURES

Calories Per Day	Play Level
25	A
50	B
75	C
100	D
150	E
200	F
250	G
300	H
400	I
500	J

PLAY PLAN A
(25 CALORIES PER DAY)

25

Choose *one* playful act *each day* from the accompanying list. These are *extra* play calories to *add* to your usual routine.

Walk a quarter-mile (3 blocks)
Cycle a mile, slowly
Swim for 3 minutes
Dance (aerobic) for 5 minutes
Clean windows for 6 minutes
Rake leaves for 6 minutes
Scrub floors for 6 minutes

Feel free to try different activities on different days.

Playful Hints . . .
• Get off to a good start — don't overdo!
• Find a playful friend!
• Don't forget — keep your play record.
• Yes — it's easy to start with, but there's lots more fun to come!

PLAY PLAN B
(50 CALORIES PER DAY)

(50)

Choose *one* playful act *each day* from the accompanying list. These are *extra* play calories to *add* to your usual routine.

Walk one-half mile
Cycle moderately for 10 minutes
Swim for 5 minutes
Dance (aerobic) for 10 minutes
Jump on a trampoline to music for 6 minutes
Hoe the garden for 10 minutes
Saw wood for 6 minutes

Insist on your play! Don't miss a day!

Playful Hints . . .

• Well done, graduation time!
• Watch out for athlete's foot, if you use changing rooms: dry your feet, and apply antifungal spray if you are prone to athlete's foot.
• Can the kids come and play with you when you walk?
• Park at the far end of the parking lot, and walk.

PLAY PLAN C
(75 CALORIES PER DAY)

(75)

Choose *one* fat-burning activity each day:

Walk at moderate speed for 15 minutes
Cycle for 15 minutes
Swim for 8 minutes
Dance (aerobic) for 12 minutes
Play table tennis for 15 minutes
Mow the lawn using a push mower for 10 minutes

Play with a friend! Do it together!

Playful Hints . . .

• Time to buy some good running shoes? Be sure they are not too tight when you try them on, with your usual socks.
• Think about some variety. Don't play the same way each day!
• Are you using your bicycle to full advantage? Should you get a bicycle?
• Play companion yet? Someone at work, on your street?

PLAY PLAN D
(100 CALORIES PER DAY)

Choose *one* activity each day and every day:

Walk at moderate speed for 20 minutes

Cycle for 18 minutes

Swim for 10 minutes

Dance (aerobic) for 15 minutes

Dance (disco) for 20 minutes

Jump on a trampoline to music for 12 minutes

Climb stairs for 8 minutes

Play table tennis for 20 minutes

Dig in the garden for 17 minutes

Saw wood for 11 minutes

Keep to your Calorie Plan!

Playful Hints . . .

• Three-figure calories! You are now four times more playful than you were three months ago!

• Is your extra play fun? It should be! If not, try some different games! Aerobic dancing? Disco dancing? Form a group!

• Take the stairs — don't wait for the elevator!

• Wear a helmet when you cycle.

PLAY PLAN E
(150 CALORIES PER DAY)

Choose *one* activity every day:

Walk at moderate speed for 30 minutes

Cycle for 25 minutes

Swim for 15 minutes

Dance (aerobic) for 25 minutes

Dance (disco) for 30 minutes

Play volleyball for 30 minutes

Play table tennis for 30 minutes

Clean windows to music for 30 minutes

Scrub floors to music for 30 minutes

Playful Hints . . .

• Do you have a companion to play with? Who do you know who would like to lose weight with you?

• Make some of your play useful: Clean windows or scrub floors to music! The exercise is burning fat.

• Think "play" whenever you have to go somewhere: Can you walk over, not ride? Is the bike handy? Why not walk to and from the restaurant? Go on, even jog a little on the way!

• If you don't drive, you won't have a parking problem (or a parking ticket).

PLAY PLAN F
(200 CALORIES PER DAY)

(200)

Walk *one mile every day* in 15 to 20 minutes

Each day *also* choose *one* other activity:

Jog slowly for 12 minutes
Cycle for 18 minutes
Swim for 10 minutes
Play racquetball for 10 minutes
Dance (aerobic) for 15 minutes
Dance (disco) for 20 minutes
Roller skate for 15 minutes
Play table tennis for 20 minutes
Rake leaves for 20 minutes
Mow the lawn for 12 minutes

Slow but sure at first if you choose to jog. And stretch.

Playful Hints . . .

• Your new fitness should start to pay dividends. Are you saving gas by walking? Mowing your own lawn?

• Have your friends and neighbors noticed your new play program? Invite them to join you! They may be envious.

• Don't forget to keep your play record.

• Take your dog on walks, he wants to play too.

PLAY PLAN G
(250 CALORIES PER DAY)

(250)

Walk *one mile every day* in 15 to 20 minutes.

Each day *also* choose *one* other activity:

Jog slowly for 18 minutes
Cycle for 26 minutes
Swim for 15 minutes
Dance (aerobic) for 24 minutes
Dance (disco) for 30 minutes
Play soccer for 20 minutes
Roller skate for 24 minutes
Jump on a trampoline to music for 18 minutes
Dig in the garden for 26 minutes
Saw wood for 15 minutes

Try new sports for variety and fun! Experience life!

Playful Hints . . .

• Have you tried roller skating? Why not give it a try for a new experience? But wear protective gear.

• What about the trampoline? Burn some more calories and have fun to music.

• Take the long way home — on foot. As you walk, you'll see things in your neighborhood you never noticed from the car.

• You have played away 2¼ pounds of fat this month!

PLAY PLAN H
(300 CALORIES PER DAY)

Walk *1½ miles every day* in 22 to 28 minutes.
Each day *also* choose one other activity:
 Jog slowly for 18 minutes
 Cycle for 26 minutes
 Swim for 15 minutes
 Dance (aerobic) for 24 minutes
 Dance (disco) for 30 minutes
 Play soccer for 20 minutes
 Roller skate for 24 minutes
 Jump on a trampoline to music for 18 minutes
 Dig in the garden for 26 minutes
 Saw wood for 15 minutes
You have now reached a desirable level of fitness and easier weight control. But you can go on!

Playful Hints . . .
• Congratulations! You are on your last Play Plan for the year.
• You have come a long way. Get yourself a good reward — and your play companion, too. How about new bicycles or some hiking boots? "His" and "Her" warm-up suits with total weight lost in one year marked on the backs.
• Keep up your stretching.
• Get plenty of variety — keep it fun!
• Celebrate!

PLAY PLAN I
(400 CALORIES PER DAY)

400

Walk *2 miles every day* in 30 to 40 minutes.
Each day *also* choose one activity:
 Jog for 20 minutes
 Cycle for 30 minutes
 Swim for 20 minutes
 Ice skate for 25 minutes
 Cross-country ski for 20 minutes
 Downhill ski for 30 minutes
 Play racquetball for 20 minutes
 Mow the lawn for 25 minutes
 Saw wood for 20 minutes
Only one play level to go!

Playful Hints . . .
• Now you are right off the charts!
• How about entering a road race — thousands do.
• If you walk, run or cycle on the roads at night, wear reflective clothing.
• Have you noticed: You are eating more but weighing less!
• Time to try some new adventures: Have you cross-country skied? Played racquetball?
• A thought for the month: Nobody said old and young cannot play together.

PLAY PLAN J
(500 CALORIES PER DAY)

Choose one activity each day:
 Walk five miles in 75 to 90 minutes
 Run for 45 minutes
 Cycle for 60 minutes
 Play racquetball for 60 minutes
 Dance (aerobic) for 60 minutes
 Play soccer for 60 minutes
 Roller skate for 65 minutes
 Mow the lawn for 60 minutes
 Saw wood for 50 minutes
This high level of fitness should be approached slowly. It involves playing vigorously for about an hour a day, or 4 percent of our 24-hour day. The player is very fit, eats a lot and has banished weight problems!

Playful Hints . . .
• Major league stuff!
• Remember, drink more water than you feel you need when it's hot.
• To avoid injuries, do your stretching exercises and vary your plan.
• You are now 20 times more playful than you were at month 1.
• You have played away 4½ pounds of fat this month!
• This level of play will keep you slim and fit forever!

References

Important sources of information relating to topics discussed in this book are arranged by chapter.

CHAPTER 1:

Bray, G.A. *Obesity in America.* U.S. Department of Health, Education and Welfare. National Institutes of Health, NIH Publication No. 79-349, 1979.

Brownell, K.K.; Stunkard, A.J. "Exercise in the Development and Control of Obesity" in Stunkard, A.J. *Obesity.* Philadelphia, W.B. Saunders, 1980.

Farquhar, John W. *The American Way of Life Need Not Be Hazardous To Your Health.* New York, W.W. Norton, 1978.

Fries, James F.; Crapo, Lawrence M. *Vitality and Aging.* San Francisco, W.H. Freeman and Company, 1981.

Storey, Rita; Cho, Margie; Scully, Ellen; Parkin, Lillie. *Popular Diets. How They Rate.* Santa Monica, Los Angeles District — California Dietetic Association, 1982.

Wood, Peter D. "Does Running Help Prevent Heart Attacks?" *Runner's World.* pp. 84-93, December 1979.

Wood, Peter D. "Physical Fitness and Sports Medicine," in *Encyclopaedia Britannica Medical and Health Annual.* pp. 286-290, 1983.

CHAPTER 2

Bennett, William; Gurin, Joel. *The Dieter's Dilemma. Eating Less and Weighing More.* New York, Basic Books, Inc., 1982.

Blair, Steven N.; Ellsworth, Nancy M.; Haskell, William L.; Stern, Michael P.; Farquhar, John W.; Wood, Peter D. "Comparison of nutrient intake in middle-aged men and women runners and controls," *Medicine and Science In Sports and Exercise.* Vol. 13 (5), pp. 310-315, 1981.

Bray, G.A. "Effect of caloric restriction on energy expenditure in obese patients," *The Lancet.* Vol. 2, pp. 397-398, 1969.

Bray, G.A. *The Obese Patient.* Philadelphia, W.B. Saunders, 1976.

Bray, G.A. (Ed.). *Obesity in America.* U.S. Department of Health, Education and Welfare. National Institutes of Health, NIH Publication No. 79-349, 1979.

Brown, J. "Nutritional and epidemiologic factors related to heart disease." in *World Review of Nutrition and Dietetics.* Vol. 12. Basel, Switzerland, S. Karger AG, 1970.

Brownell, K.D.; Stunkard, A.J. "Exercise in the development and control of obesity." in Stunkard, A.J. (Ed), *Obesity.* Philadelphia, W.B. Saunders, 1980.

Epstein, L.; Miller, G.J.; Stitt, F.W.; Morris, J.N. "Vigorous exercise in leisure time, coronary risk factors, and resting electrocardiogram in middle-aged male civil servants," *British Medical Journal.* Vol. 38, pp. 403-409, 1976.

Garrow, J.S. *Energy Balance and Obesity in Man* (2nd Edition). Amsterdam, Elsevier, 1978.

Gordon, Tavia; Kagan, Abraham; Garcia-Palmieri, Mario; Kannel, William B.; Zukel, William J.; Tillotson, Jeanne; Sorlie, Paul; Hjortland, Marthana. "Diet and its relation to coronary heart disease and death in three populations," *Circulation.* Vol. 63 (3), pp. 500-515, 1981.

Gwinup, G. "Effect of exercise alone on the weight of obese women," *Archives of Internal Medicine.* Vol. 135, pp. 676-680, 1975.

Katahn, Martin. *The 200 Calorie Solution.* New York, W.W. Norton and Company, 1982.

Mayer, J.; Roy, P.; Miltra, K.P. "Relation between caloric intake, body weight and physical work; studies in industrial male population in West Bengal," *American Journal of Clinical Nutrition.* Vol. 4, p. 169, 1956.

McArdle, W.D.; Katch, F.K.; Katch, V.L. *Exercise Physiology: Energy, Nutrition, and Human Performance.* Philadelphia, Lea and Febiger, 1981.

Thompson, J.K.; Jarvie, G.J.; Lahey, B.B.; Cureton, K.J. "Exercise and obesity: Etiology, physiology and intervention," *Psychological Bulletin.* Vol. 91, pp. 55-79, 1982.

Van Itallie, T.B.; "Dietary approaches to the treatment of obesity," *Psychiatric Clinics of North America.* Vol. 1, pp. 609-620, 1978.

Vodak, P.A.; Wood, P.D.; Haskell, W.L.; Williams, P.T. "HDL-cholesterol and other plasma lipid and lipoprotein concentrations in middle-aged male and female tennis players," *Metabolism.* Vol. 29, pp. 745-752, 1980.

White, Philip L.; Mondeika, Therese. *Diet and Exercise: Synergism in Health Maintenance.* Chicago, American Medical Association, 1982.

Wood, Peter D.; Haskell, William L.; Blair, Steven N.; Williams, Paul T.; Krauss, Ronald M.; Lindgren, Frank T.; Albers, John J.; Ho, Ping H.; Farquhar, John W. "Increased exercise level and plasma lipoprotein concentrations: A one-year, randomized, controlled study in sedentary, middle-aged men," *Metabolism,* Vol. 32(1), pp. 31-39, 1983.

CHAPTER 3:

Metropolitan Life Insurance Company, New York. "New Weight Standards for Men and Women," *Statistical Bulletin.* (Nov-Dec), 1959.

CHAPTER 4:

Fries, James F.; Crapo, Lawrence M. *Vitality and Aging.* San Francisco, W.H. Freeman and Company, 1981.

CHAPTER 5:

Sheehan, George A. *Running and Being. The Total Experience.* New York, Simon and Schuster, 1978.

CHAPTER 6:

American College of Sports Medicine. *Sports Injuries: An Aid to Prevention and Treatment.* (From American College of Sports Medicine, 1440 Monroe St., Madison, WI 53706.)

Conrad, C. Carson. *How Different Sports Rate In Promoting Physical Fitness.* President's Council on Physical Fitness and Sports, Washington, D.C., U.S. Department of Health, Education and Welfare, Public Health Service, February 1979.

Cooper, Kenneth H. *The New Aerobics.* New York, Bantam Books, 1970.

D'Ambrosia, R.; Drez, D. *Prevention and Treatment of Running Injuries.* Thorofare, New Jersey, Charles B. Slack, Inc., 1982.

Thompson, Paul D.; Funk, Erik J.; Carleton, Richard A.; Sturner, William Q. "Incidence of Death During Jogging in Rhode Island from 1975 through 1980," *Journal of the American Medical Association.* Vol. 247(18), pp. 2535-2538, (May), 1982.

Wood, Peter D. *Run To Health.* New York, Charter Books, 1980.

CHAPTER 7:
(No references for this chapter)

CHAPTER 8:

American Heart Association. *Heart Facts.* Dallas, 1983. (From American Heart Association, National Center, 7320 Greenville Ave., Dallas, TX 75231.)

Bjorntorp, P. "Physical Training in the Treatment of Obesity," *International Journal of Obesity.* Vol. 2, pp. 149-151, 1978.

Doll, Richard; Peto, Richard. *The Causes of Cancer.* Oxford, Oxford University Press, 1981.

Gilmore, C.P. *Exercising for Fitness.* Alexandria, Virginia, Time-Life Books, 1981.

Gordon, Tavia; Kagan, Abraham; Garcia-Palmieri, Mario; Kannel, William B.; Zukel, William J.; Tillotson, Jeanne; Sorlie, Paul; Hjortland, Marthana. "Diet and its relation to coronary heart disease and death in three populations," *Circulation.* Vol. 63(3), pp. 500-515, 1981.

Gwinup, G. "Effect of Exercise Alone on the Weight of Obese Women," *Archives of Internal Medicine.* Vol. 135, pp. 676-680, May 1975.

Hartung, G.H.; Foreyt, J.P.; Mitchell, R.E. "Relation of Diet to High-Density Lipoprotein Cholesterol in Middle-Aged Marathon Runners, Joggers, and Inactive Men," *New England Journal of Medicine.* Vol. 302(7), pp. 357-361, Feb 1980.

Kostrubala, Thaddeus. *The Joy of Running.* New York, J.B. Lippincott Company, 1976.

Kramsch, Dieter M.; Aspen, Anita J.; Abramowitz, Bruce M.; Kreimendahl, Toby; Hood, William B., Jr. "Reduction of Coronary Atherosclerosis by Moderate Conditioning Exercise in Monkeys on an Atherogenic Diet," *New England Journal of Medicine.* Vol. 305(25), pp. 1483-1489, December 1981.

Milvy, P. "The Marathon: Physiological, Medical, Epidemiological Studies," *Annals of the New York Academy of Sciences.* Vol. 301, 1977.

Morris, J.N.; Chave, S.P.W.; Adam, C.; Sirey, C.; Epstein, L.; Sheehan, D.J. "Vigorous Exercise in Leisure-Time and the Incidence of Coronary Heart Disease," *The Lancet.* Vol. 1, pp. 333-339, February 1973.

Morris, J.N.; Kagan, A.; Pattison, D.C.; Gardner, M.J.; Raffle,

P.A.B. "Incidence and Prediction of Ischaemic Heart Disease in London Busmen," *The Lancet.* Vol. 2, pp. 553-559, September 1966.

Paffenbarger, R.S., Jr.; Laughlin, M.E.; Gima, A.S.; Black, R.A. "Work Activity of Longshoremen as Related to Death from Coronary Heart Disease and Stroke," *New England Journal of Medicine.* Vol. 282(20), pp. 1109-1114, May 1970.

Paffenbarger, R.S., Jr.; Wing, A.L.; Hyde, R.T. "Physical Activity as an Index of Heart Attack Risk in College Alumni," *American Journal of Epidemiology.* Vol. 108(3), pp. 161-175, September 1978.

Pollock, Michael L.; Wilmore, Jack H.; Fox, Samuel M. III. *Health and Fitness Through Physical Activity.* New York, John Wiley and Sons, 1978.

Sheehan, George A. *Running and Being. The Total Experience.* New York, Simon and Schuster, 1978.

Stalonas, P.M.; Johnson, W.G.; Christ, M. "Behavior Modification for Obesity: The Evaluation of Exercise, Contingency Management, and Program Adherence," *Consulting and Clinical Psychology.* Vol. 46(3), pp. 463-469, 1978.

Wood, Peter D. "Does Running Help Prevent Heart Attacks?" *Runner's World.* pp. 84-93, December 1979.

Wood, Peter D. *Run To Health.* New York, Charter Books, 1980.

Wood, Peter D. "Smoking and Running. Can the Two Addictions Co-Exist?" *Runner's World.* pp. 80-83, September 1979.

Wood, Peter D. "The Eat-More, Weigh-Less Diet," *Runner's World.* pp. 42-44, September 1980.

Wood, Peter D.; Haskell, William L.; Blair, Steven N.; Williams, Paul T.; Krauss, Ronald M.; Lindgren, Frank T.; Albers, John J.; Ho, Ping H.; Farquhar, John W. "Increased Exercise Level And Plasma Lipoprotein Concentrations: A One-Year, Randomized, Controlled Study In Sedentary, Middle-Aged Men," *Metabolism.* Vol. 32(1), pp. 31-39, 1983.

Wood, Peter D.; Haskell, William L. "The Effect of Exercise on Plasma High Density Lipoproteins," *Lipids.* Vol. 14(4), pp. 417-427, April 1979.

Wood, Peter D.; Haskell, William L.; Stern, Michael P.; Lewis, Steven; Perry, Christopher. "Plasma Lipoprotein Distributions in Male and Female Runners," *Annals of the New York Academy of Sciences.* Vol. 301, pp. 748-762, 1977.

CHAPTER 9

American Heart Association. *Diet and Coronary Disease.* Dallas, 1978. (From American Heart Association, National Center, 7320 Greenville Ave., Dallas, TX 75231).

Blair, Steven N.; Ellsworth, Nancy M.; Haskell, William L.; Stern, Michael P.; Farquhar, John W.; Wood, Peter D. "Comparison of Nutrient Intake in Middle-Aged Men and Women Runners and Controls," *Medicine and Science in Sports and Exercise.* Vol. 13(5), pp. 310-315, 1981.

Brody, Jane E. *Jane Brody's Nutrition Book. A Lifetime Guide to Good Eating for Better Health and Weight Control.* New York, W.W. Norton and Company, 1981.

Committee on Dietary Allowances, Food and Nutrition Board, National Research Council. *Recommended Dietary Allowances,* Ninth Revised Edition, 1980. Washington, D.C., National Academy of Sciences, 1980.

Dietary Intake Findings, United States, 1971-74. Data from the National Health and Nutrition Examination Survey. DHEW Publication No. (HRA) 77-1647, 1977.

Doll, Richard; Peto, Richard. *The Causes of Cancer.* Oxford, Oxford University Press, 1981.

Food and Nutrition Intake of Individuals in One Day in the United States, Spring 1977. USDA Nationwide Food Consumption Survey, 1977-78. Preliminary Report No. 2, 1980.

Gordon, Tavia; Fisher, Marian; Ernst, Nancy; Rifkind, Basil M. "Relation of Diet to LDL Cholesterol, VLDL Cholesterol and Triglycerides in White Adults. The Lipid Research Clinics Prevalence Study," *Arteriosclerosis.* Vol. 2(6), pp. 502-512, November-December, 1982.

Lappé, Frances Moore. *Diet for a Small Planet.* 2nd Edition. New York, Ballantine, 1975.

Mason, Dean T.; Guthrie, Helen. *The Medicine Called Nutrition.* Englewood Cliffs, New Jersey, Best Foods - A Unit of CPC North America, 1979.

Pritikin, Nathan. *The Pritikin Permanent Weight-Loss Manual.* New York, Bantam Books, 1981.

Robertson, Laurel; Flinders, Carol; Godfrey, Bronwen; *Laurel's Kitchen.* Berkeley, California, Nilgiri Press, 1976.

Select Committee on Nutrition and Human Needs, United States Senate. *Dietary Goals for the United States,* 2nd Edition. Washington, D.C., U.S. Government Printing Office, 1977.

U.S. Department of Agriculture; U.S. Department of Health, Education and Welfare; *Nutrition and Your Health. Dietary Guidelines for Americans.* Home and Garden Bulletin No. 232.

U.S. Department of Health, Education, and Welfare, Public Health Service, Office of the Assistant Secretary for Health and Surgeon General. *Healthy People: The Surgeon General's Report on Health Promotion and Disease Prevention, 1979.* DHEW Publication No. (PHS) 79-55071. Washington, D.C., U.S. Government Printing Office, 1979.

Wood, P.D.; Haskell, W.L.; Terry, R.B.; Ho, P.H.; Blair, S.N. "Effects of a Two-Year Running Program on Plasma Lipoproteins, Body Fat and Dietary Intake in Initially Sedentary Men" (Abstract), *Medicine and Science in Sports and Exercise.* Vol. 14(2), p. 104, 1982.

CHAPTER 10

Brody, Jane E. *Jane Brody's Nutrition Book. A Lifetime Guide to Good Eating for Better Health and Weight Control.* New York, W.W. Norton and Company, 1981.

Burkitt, D.P. "Large-Bowel Cancer: An Epidemiological Jigsaw Puzzle," *Journal National Cancer Institute.* Vol. 54, pp. 3-6, 1975.

Council for Agricultural Science and Technology (CAST); *Diet, Nutrition and Cancer: A Critique.* Special Publication No. 13, 1982 (from the Council for Agricultural Science and Technology, Iowa State University, Ames, IA 50011).

Doll, Richard; Peto, Richard. *The Causes of Cancer.* Oxford, Oxford University Press, 1981.

Food and Nutrition Board, National Research Council. *Toward Healthful Diets.* Washington, D.C., National Academy of Sciences, 1980.

Kay, Ruth McPherson. "Dietary Fiber," *Journal of Lipid Research.* Vol. 23(2), pp. 221-242, February 1982.

Kromhout, D.; Bosschieter, E.B.; De Lezenne Coulander, C. "Dietary Fiber and 10-Year Mortality From Coronary Heart Disease, Cancer, and All Causes," *The Lancet.* Vol. 2, pp. 518-522, September 1982.

Lappé, Frances Moore. *Diet For A Small Planet.* 2nd Edition. New York, Ballantine, 1975.

National Research Council. *Diet, Nutrition, and Cancer.* Washington, D.C., National Academy Press, 1982.

Painter, N.S.; Burkitt, D.P. "Diverticular Disease of the Colon: A Deficiency Disease of Western Civilization," *British Medical Journal.* Vol. 2, pp. 450-454, 1971.

Rivlin, Richard S. "Nutrition and Cancer: State of the Art Relationship of Several Nutrients to the Development of Cancer," *Journal of the American College of Nutrition.* Vol. 1, pp. 75-88, 1982.

Robertson, Laurel; Flinders, Carol; Godfrey, Bronwen. *Laurel's Kitchen.* Berekeley, California, Nilgiri Press, 1976.

Select Committee on Nutrition and Human Needs, United States Senate. *Dietary Goals for the United States,* 2nd Edition. Washington, D.C., U.S. Government Printing Office, 1977.

CHAPTER 11

Anitschkow, N.; "Uber die Veranderungen der Kaninchenaorta bei experimenteller Cholesterinsteatose," *Beitrage zur Pathologischen Anatomie.* Vol. 56, p. 379, 1913.

Baboriak, Joseph J.; Anderson, Alfred J.; Hoffmann, Raymond G. "Smoking, Alcohol and Coronary Artery Occlusion," *Atherosclerosis.* Vol. 43, pp. 277-282, 1982.

Blackwelder, W.C.; Yano, K.; Rhoads, G.G.; Kagan, A.; Gorton, T.; Palesch, Y. "Alcohol and Morality: The Honolulu Heart Study," *American Journal Medicine.* Vol. 68, p. 164, 1980.

Brody, Jane E. *Jane Brody's Nutrition Book. A Lifetime Guide to Good Eating for Better Health and Weight Control.* New York, W.W. Norton and Company, 1981.

Gruchow, Harvey W.; Hoffman, Raymond G.; Anderson, Alfred J.; Barboriak, Joseph J. "Effects of Drinking Patterns on the Relationship Between Alcohol and Coronary Occulsion," *Atherosclerosis.* Vol. 43, pp. 393-404, 1982.

Myant, N.B. *The Biology of Cholesterol and Related Steroids.* London, William Heinemann Medical Books Ltd, 1981.

Schottenfeld, D. "Alcohol As a Co-Factor in the Etiology of Cancer," *British Medical Journal.* Vol. 1, p. 1483, 1978.

Select Committee on Nutrition and Human Needs, United States Senate. *Dietary Goals for the United States,* 2nd Edition. Washington, D.C., U.S. Government Printing Office, 1977.

Yano, K.; Rhoads, G.G.; Kagan, A. "Coffee, Alcohol, and Risk of Coronary Heart Disease Among Japanese Men Living in Hawaii," *New England Journal of Medicine.* Vol. 297, p. 405, 1977.

CHAPTER 12

Blanton, Parke; California Agriculture Directory 1982-83. Sacramento, California, California Service Agency, 1982.

The Packer's Produce Availability and Merchandising Guide. Annual magazine publication of the weekly National Fresh Fruit and Vegetable Industry Newspaper (*The Packer*). Vol. 89(53), 1982.

ABOUT THE AUTHOR

Dr. Peter Wood is a Professor of Medicine (Research) at Stanford University and Deputy Director of the Stanford Heart Disease Prevention Program. He is a member of the American Institute of Nutrition and of the American Society of Clinical Nutrition. Dr. Wood is also a fellow of the Arteriosclerosis Council and the Epidemiology Council of the American Heart Association.

Dr. Wood's scientific articles have appeared in medical journals around the world. He has written for *The New York Times* and *The New York Times Magazine*, and is the Science Editor of *Runner's World* magazine.

Educated in England, Dr. Wood worked in Canada, Australia and New Zealand as a research chemist before moving to California in 1962. He lives at Stanford, California, with his wife Christine.